YOGA SECRETS FOR EXTRAORDINARY HEALTH AND LONG LIFE

FRANK RUDOLPH YOUNG

YOGA SECRETS FOR EXTRAORDINARY HEALTH AND LONG LIFE.

For more information please visit:

www.parkerpub.co

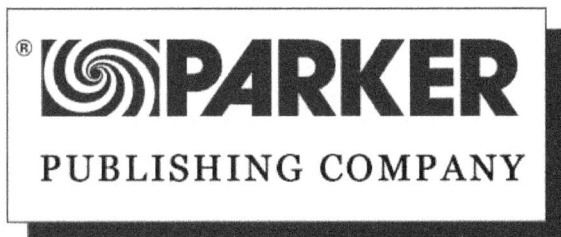

PARKER
PUBLISHING COMPANY

parkerpub.co

*This book is dedicated to the secret Yogis,
to my medical and dental ancestors,
to chiropractic and other natural systems of healing, and to the thousands
of patients and volunteers on several continents, both mine & theirs who
made it possible.*

YOGA SECRETS FOR EXTRAORDINARY HEALTH AND LONG LIFE

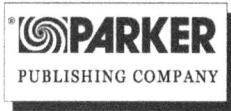

PARKER

PUBLISHING COMPANY

1

How Yoga Can Bring You
the Flexible Spine of a Young Person

Using Superior Body Mechanics to Conquer
the Clutch of Gravity

A. *How Yoga specifically helps you.* Yoga mov-asanas (moving postures) will bring you miracle health by overcoming The Four Natural Health Wreckers which ruin you from without and within. These are:

1. The Clutch of Gravity on You
2. The Tortures of Your Conscious Thinking
3. Your Volcanic Emotions
4. Your Bio-Cosmic Instability

In one way or another, these four health villains undermine you every moment of the day, convert you into an inferior person, age you prematurely, and shorten your life markedly. But you can resist their scourges amazingly with Yoga mov-asanas.

B. *How the Clutch of Gravity on You Ruins Your Life.* The incessant downpull of gravity on you alters your anatomy, your physiology, and your mental and psychic responses. Over thousands of years, due to mankind's two-legged stance, gravity has altered your inherited skeletal structure. Most of the stress of gravity on you is borne by the inter-vertebral discs of your balancing spine. These are the 24 small pads of fibrous cartilage which are sandwiched between every pair of your 24 vertebrae. They act as shock absorbers against every strain and stress on your spinal column.

But your intervertebral discs (also called "spinal discs") shrink with age and use. During your lifetime you may lose a total of three to four

13

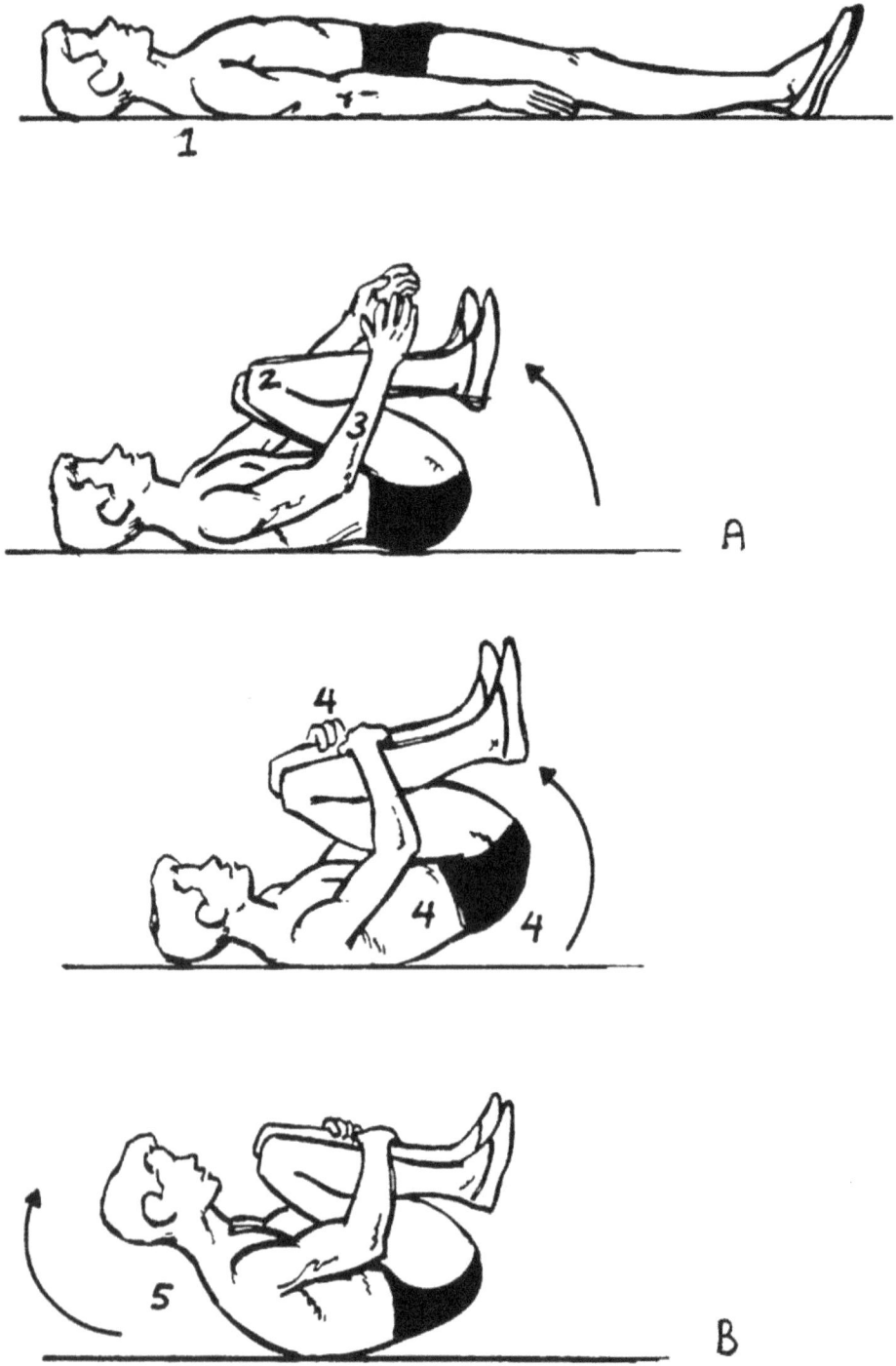

Figure 1
The Resting Back Arch

inches or more in height. If you could delay the "death-dealing shrinking" of your intervertebral discs about 25 percent, you could live considerably longer, look much younger, feel much taller and stronger, overcome disease more easily, and be far more fascinating to others. The Yoga mov-asana to delay the death-dealing shrinking of your invertebral discs is The Resting Back Arch, described as follows. (Follow Figure 1.)

Lifting Pressure from Your Spinal Nerves with the Resting Back Arch

The position to assume (Figure 1A)

1. Lie flat on your back.
2. Bend your knees and flex them to your chest.
3. Clasp them with your arms.

How to do this Yoga mov-asana (Figure 1B)

4. Exhale and clasp your knees so tightly with your arms that your hips rise several inches off the floor or your bed. (You will feel a strong pull all through the lower two-thirds of your back.) At the same time,

5. Raise your head slightly off the ground and stretch it away from your body. (You will feel a strong pull all the way through your neck and the upper part of your back).

Frequency: 10 times. 1 set (group of repetitions). Once a day.

What the Resting Back Arch does for you:

1. By stretching your whole back and neck, it widens the space between your vertebrae, where your *inter*-vertebral discs lie. This encourages your shrinking intervertebral discs to stop shrinking and to thicken again, instead.

2. It firms the muscles of your waist and flattens your abdomen.

3. By firming the muscles of your waist, it also squeezes your liver and spleen, massages your stomach, and forces fecal matter down your bowels, combatting constipation.

4. It limbers your back, not in the dangerous backward bending direction, which can wear down your intervertebral discs and even cause you to suffer a "slipped disc," but in the safe, *forward bending* direction.

5. The nerves in your back will be relieved of much of the compression of your packed-down vertebrae and restore the circulation of your organs closer to normal level. You will live considerably longer as a result. And you will look

much younger and be far more physically attractive, feel much younger and stronger, and overcome disease more easily. It multiplies concentration power.

How Yoga Helped Thelma R. Move Like a Young Girl

Thelma R. felt increasingly as if her spine were being hammered down into a shorter column. An aging numbness seemed to pervade her back, from waist to neck. The impulsive drive of youth left her. Her life had been wasted, she grieved. She had been a "work horse." Now she was turning into an "old horse," too.

Since her physician's diagnosis revealed nothing clinically wrong with Thelma's back, I taught her the Yoga mov-asana, The Resting Back Arch. A week later she looked an inch taller. Her eyes sparkled, and she smiled readily. A month later she seemed nearly two inches taller because the shape of her torso had changed. In six weeks she regained the flexibility of a young woman. "I am going to make up for lost time!" she cried. "I feel like a young girl again!"

Special Yoga Breathing to Expand Your Rib Cage (Your Solar Breath)

When your rib box shrinks to smaller than it should be, your heart cannot do its best job, no matter how wisely you eat, exercise, or think. Your heart requires room to enlarge when your blood fills it. If the room is limited, your heart has to push the neighboring structures out of its way. But since your heart cannot push your rib box out of its way, it overenlarges (hypertrophies) in its vain effort to do so. But that enlargement thickens its own wall and reduces the space for blood within its own chambers. So, the amount of oxygen-carrying blood that can pass through it is diminished in those two ways, and your body cells and your brain receive less life-giving oxygen to carry on your life functions. Solve this impasse by expanding your rib cage. The secret Yoga mov-asana for it is Your Solar Breath. Here is how to do it. (Follow Figure 2.)

How to Do the Solar Breath mov-asana

1. Sit comfortably in a straight chair, hands resting, palms down, on your thighs. (Figure 2A).

2. Start breathing at 2 (Figure 2B), way down deep.

3. Expand the breathing to 3,4,5,6 (Figure 2B), until your rib box is popping from front to back, and from side to side.

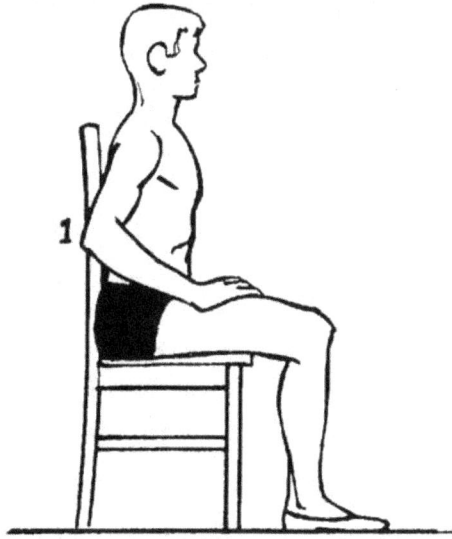

A

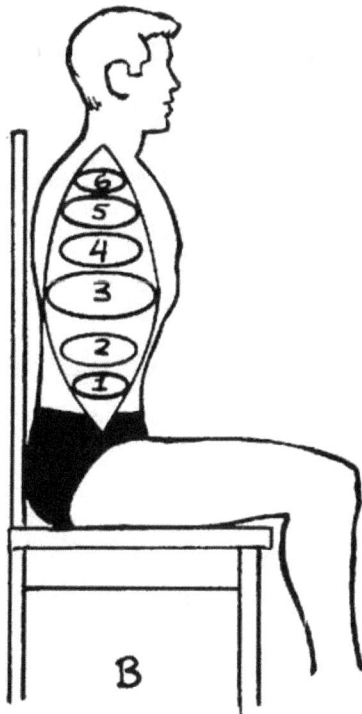

B

Figure 2
Your Solar Breath

4. Don't hold your breath when your rib box is "popping." *Exhale* then, instead.

Frequency: 2 repetitions. 2 sets (groups of repetitions) a day. 5 times a week.

What Your Solar Breath mov-asana does for you:

1. Develops your breathing muscles and helps your heart and lungs to function more efficiently.

2. Increases the height of your rib box, thereby elevating your breasts.

3. Your higher rib box permits more energy with *prana* (oxygen) to be carried in your blood to your brain. That increases the voltage of the nerve-electricity which your brain discharges into your body. Your superior at work feels surer of you. You think sharper and with more originality.

4. Stimulates the vertebrae halfway up on your upper back (your 4-5 dorsals). Stimulates also those vertebrae by your waistline (your twelfth dorsal). All these improve your aorta, heart, and bladder. They also relax your visceral spasms, such as those of the far end of your stomach, and of your duodenum, the small intestine into which your stomach passes your partially-digested food.

How Bill E. Added Many Years of Health to His Life

Bill E. was easily winded, so he avoided physical competition. He caught chest colds "like nothing" and they clung to him a long time. His pulse was faster than average, and his heart beat was not hard and thumping. His chest was flat, too, and deprived him of the "husky" look he wanted. He resigned himself to the conclusion that he was frail by nature, and doomed to a comparatively short life.

I taught Bill the secret of His Solar Breath. He couldn't believe it as his chest rose higher and higher, day by day. In two months his rib box was popping from front to back, and from side to side. People remarked that he was getting "big and chesty." He felt more dynamic, too, for his tissues received more oxygen, and his heart had more pumping room.

Bill felt the increased voltage of nerve-electricity which his brain flashed now into his body. He no longer viewed himself as being frail by nature and felt that he had added years to his life. He started competing in the physical contests he enjoyed and was surprisingly good in them.

Restoring Your Spinal Column Flexibility
to Relax Your Back Muscles

When your back muscles are chronically tense they limit the flexibility of your spine. The supply of nerve-electricity to your other muscles is reduced, too, and waste products accumulate in all of them and reduce their tone. Your muscles then require a greater-than-normal charge of nerve-electricity to stimulate them into normal action. When your muscles don't receive that charge, you lose body tone and are under par physically and mentally. You feel lackadaisical, easily fatigued, out-of-sorts, and antisocial. You lose your ability to draw people to you and make them like you. But there is an easy Yoga mov-asana to overcome back muscle tension by flushing the stagnated blood out of them. It is The Yoga Back Curl. Here is how to do it. (Follow Figure 3.)

The position to assume (Figures 3 A,B)

1. Lie face down, relaxed, with your legs straight, heels together.
2. Straighten your arms by your sides, palms down.
3. Point your toes backwards.

How to do this Yoga mov-asana (Figure 3 C)

4. Keep your arms and knees straight.
5. Inhale, and raise your arms—and your legs—*at the same time.*
6. *Keep your arms and legs straight*, remember, with your *palms down*, and your *toes pointed backwards.*
7. Raise your head, too. At the same time,
8. (Not shown in figure.) Visualize yourself as being *the most favored person on earth.*
9. Hold the position (and the visualization) for two seconds.
10. Then exhale and relax.

Frequency: 7 times. 2 sets (groups of repetitions). 4 times a week.

What the Yoga Back Curl does for you:

1. Strengthens the muscles that keep your back straight (your sacrospinalis, or spinal erector muscles).
2. With a straighter back you feel taller and look more fashionable. You feel more confident, more appreciated, more sure of yourself.
3. You infect others with this attitude, and they delight in seeing you.
4. Without your even suspecting it, you start drawing to you swiftly the best things in life. You think faster, more flexibly, and create easier.
5. You relieve muscular micro-spasms in your back and help renormalize the alignments of your different vertebrae.

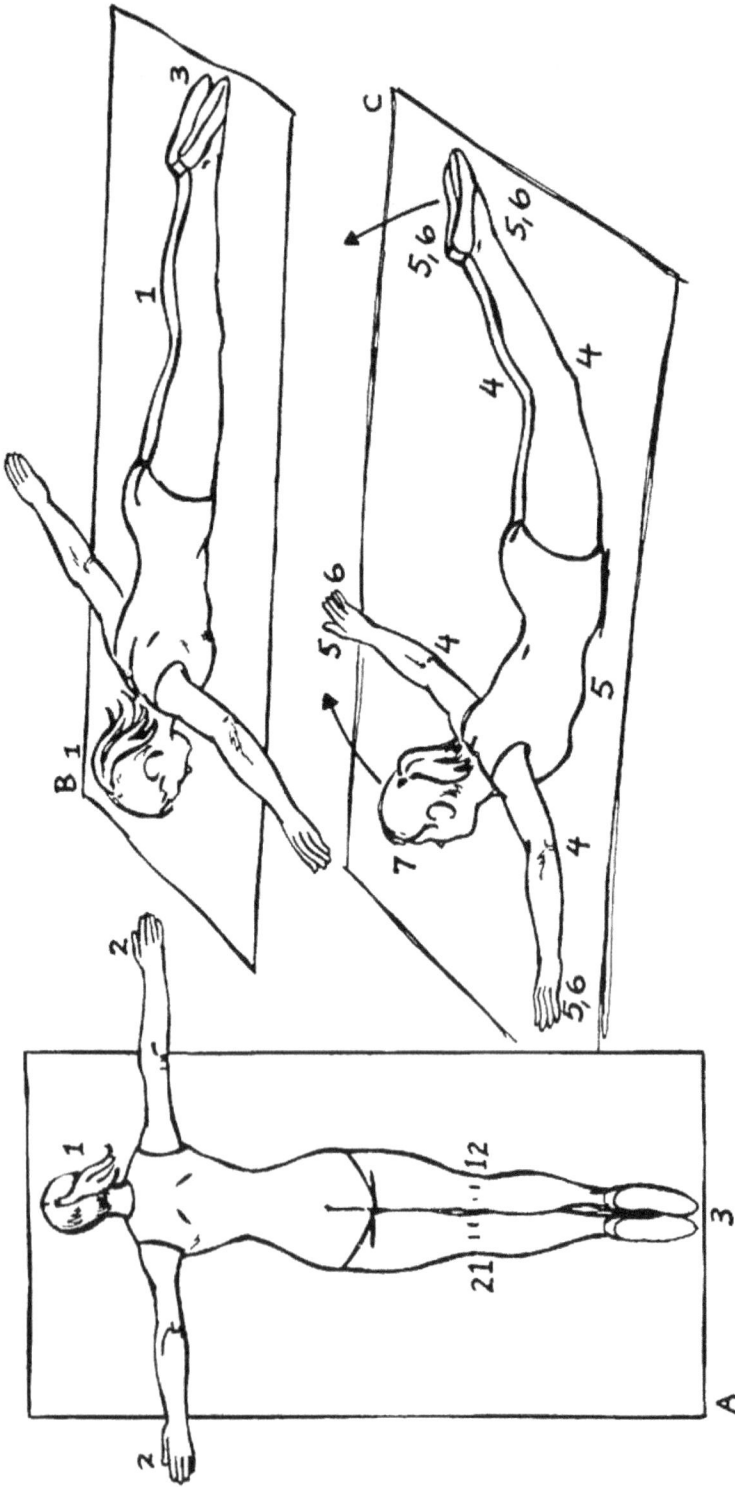

Figure 3
The Yoga Back Curl

How Lena N. Relieved Her Lower "Backaches"

Lena N. had nothing wrong organically that showed up in a clinic examination. But her lower back "plagued" her, particularly whenever she was up and active for hours, and thoroughly spoiled her business and social life. Sedatives and a brace from her orthopedist relieved the condition, but she refused these after a while. Chiropractic adjustments helped her, too, but not permanently. Her trouble seemed to be mainly postural. As the day wore on, her back muscles tired, and her nerve pains supersensitized. Then the cosmic forces of noises, vibrations, telepathic influences, the presence of others, different colors, environments, etc., disturbed her physiology and routed her natural personality.

I taught Lena the Yoga mov-asana to restore the flexibility of her spinal column and relax her back muscles. In a week she strengthened her spinal erector (her spine-straightening) muscles enough to feel taller and look more fashionable. By visualizing this new picture of herself as she did this mov-asana, she at once felt more appreciated and more sure of herself. Her mental alertness stunned people.

Her lower back "bothered" her far less during the day thereafter, and she infected others with her new attitude. Without even suspecting it, she drew to her the best things in life. Six months later, through the influence of her boss, she was offered an important position in *another* firm. She was so changed that the vice-president of the new firm fell in love with her at sight, and married her within a year.

Regulating Your Bio-Cosmic Instability

Vast cosmic tides which no man controls directly can kill living organisms through relatively minute changes in temperature. The greater your sensitivity, the more destructive these shocks are to you, and the more your whole life is twisted out of shape . . . your spine included.

These vast cosmic tides are set into motion by the planets of the Zodiac. They create in you wide undulations of mood and physiological well-being. Noted examples are: the lunar rhythms which (if you are a woman) seem directly related to your ovulation cycle; the full moon, which seems related to your mental balance; and rainy weather, which seems related to the electron charges in your body, and hence, to the power of your nerve-electricity.

The cosmic forces of the Zodiac affect your cells physiologically. They alter the responses of your glands and sympathetic nervous system to your environment, and these create tensions in you which contract certain muscles, especially those of your spine. You are altered into a different kind of person, just as you are quite different at 10 A.M. from what you are at 10 P.M. It is one of the primary causes of your premature aging, for your body over-exerts itself to survive those merciless planetary pulls.

The effective Yoga mov-asana to fight back these pulls is Your Torso Trimmer. It regulates your bio-cosmic instability and greatly retards your aging. It draws (or stretches) your upper body "away" from your lower body, so to speak, preventing the vast cosmic tides from throwing your muscles into spasms through their effects on your brain. Here is how to do it. (Follow Figure 4.)

Preventing Aging Through a Yoga Mov-asana— Your Torso Trimmer

The position to assume (Figure 4A)

1. Stand with heels 10 to 14 inches apart, depending on your height, feet pointing normally slightly outwards,

2. Arms hanging loosely at your sides.

How to do this Yoga mov-asana (Figure 4 B,C)

3. Inhale and twist body to left. At the same time

4. Bend right arm and cross it above your head. Also

5. Bend *left* arm and cross it behind your lower back. Exhale.

6. Then inhale and reverse the movement. That is (Figure 4 C),

7. Inhale and twist body to right. At the same time,

8. Raise bent *left* arm and cross it above your head. Simultaneously,

9. Lower bent *right* arm and cross it behind your lower back.

10. Repeat the simple mov-asana from side-to-side. Keep the motion continuous, like that of a ballet dancer, and with rhythm and energy. Cross your arms far over your head and behind your back. Let your upper arm stretch the sides of your back, and your lower arm stretch your shoulders.

Frequency: 8 repetitions. 1-2 sets (groups of repetitions). 4 times a week.

What Your Torso Trimmer does for you (Figure 4D)

1. Shaves off the bulges on the sides of your upper back and replaces them with youthful lines.

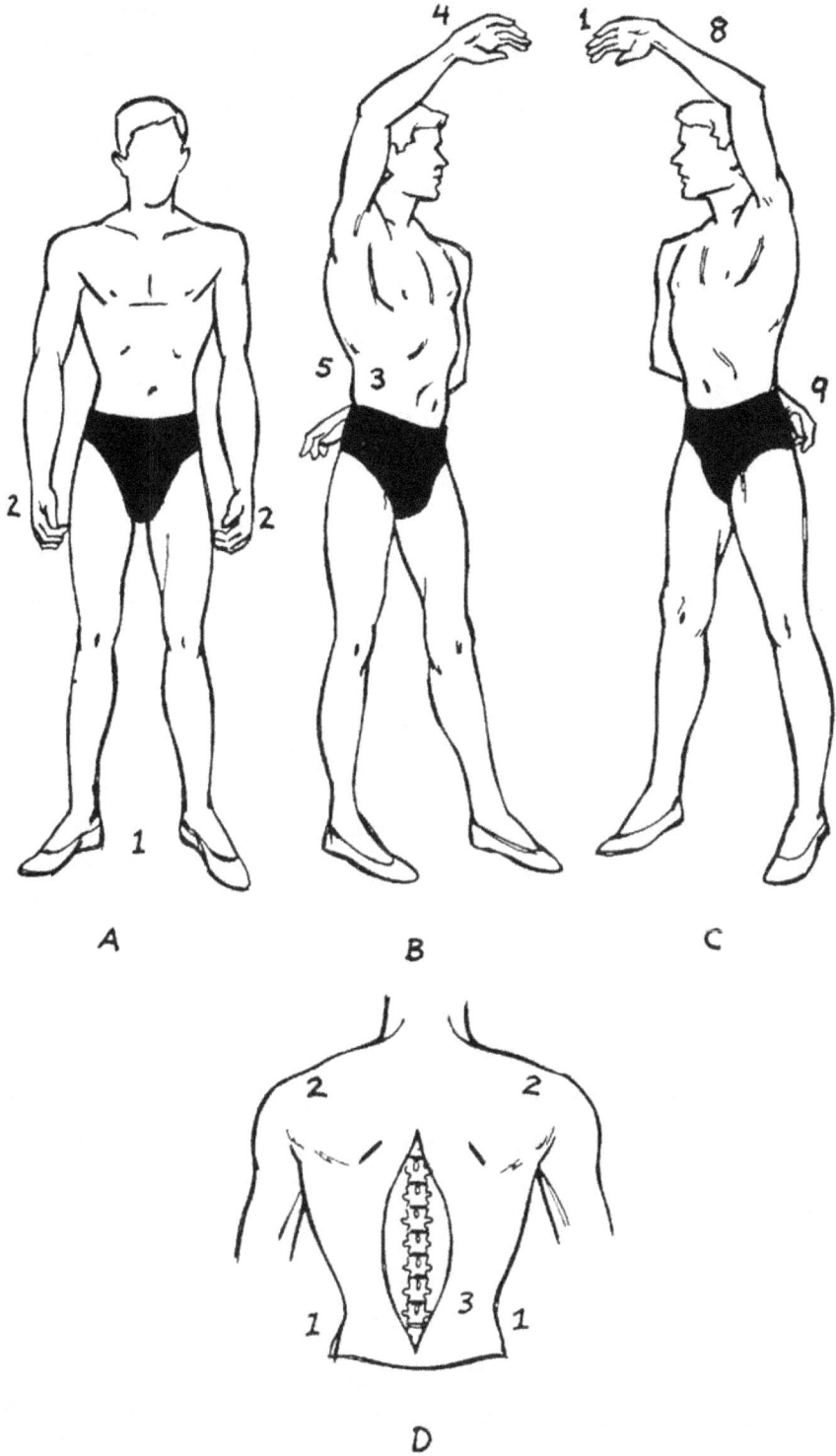

A   B   C

D
Figure 4
Your Torso Trimmer

2. Brings flexibility to your shoulder joints to prevent and combat bursitis.

3. Stimulates the vertebrae around your waist (your tenth, eleventh, and twelfth dorsals, and your 1-2 lumbars). This improves the functions of your pancreas, adrenals, spleen, colon, bladder. It aids the muscles that overlie the spinal nerves which supply these organs with nerve-electricity, preventing cosmic tides from throwing them into spasms. Such "visceral freedom" permits more blood to feed your brain and improve its thinking power.

How Norman L. and His Wife Felt and Looked Youthful Again

Norman L. and his wife, Joan, were middle-aged. They did not relish exercise, but their upper backs were acquiring the unflattering buffalo-look of the aging person with habitual bad posture. It added from ten to 15 years to their apparent ages. Norman and his wife tried different corrective exercises, but found them boring, unusually fatiguing to their little-used muscles, or too time-consuming.

I taught them Their Torso Trimmer mov-asana. Its simple side-to-side movement, like that of a ballet dancer's, delighted them, and they did it with rhythm and vigor. They felt it smoothing off the fat bulges on the sides of their upper backs and replacing them with sensations of trimness and flexibility. As a bonus benefit, Norman's wife, Joan, even felt her shoulder joints turn limber and lose the stiffness of her chronic bursitis. Their very minds limbered with ideas, too.

Three months later, the two of them looked like different people. They "appeared" taller and excitably fashionable, as if 20 years younger.

Effect of The Yoga Circadian Shock Nullifier

I discovered the bio-rhythm as early as 1945, and taught and published it in *Solar Diet* (pp. 12-13) in 1954, or from ten to 17 years ahead of science! I called it "Rhythm Regularity." Rhythm Regularity means that your different physiological (circadian) rhythms fluctuate daily and alter your resistance or vulnerability to drugs, stress, allergy, pain, and infection. These circadian rhythms are:

your activity-sleep rhythm

your urine excretion rhythm

your menstrual rhythm (if you are a woman)

your body temperature rhythm

your potassium excretion rhythm

your sodium chloride (salt) excretion rhythm

your calcium excretion rhythm

your rectal temperature rhythm

Each rhythm, when it fluctuates "wrongly" during the day, subjects your cells to a "circadian shock" that reduces your physiological voltage. The secret Yoga mov-asana to nullify this debilitating daily change in you when it occurs is Your Circadian Shock Nullifier. (Follow Figure 5.)

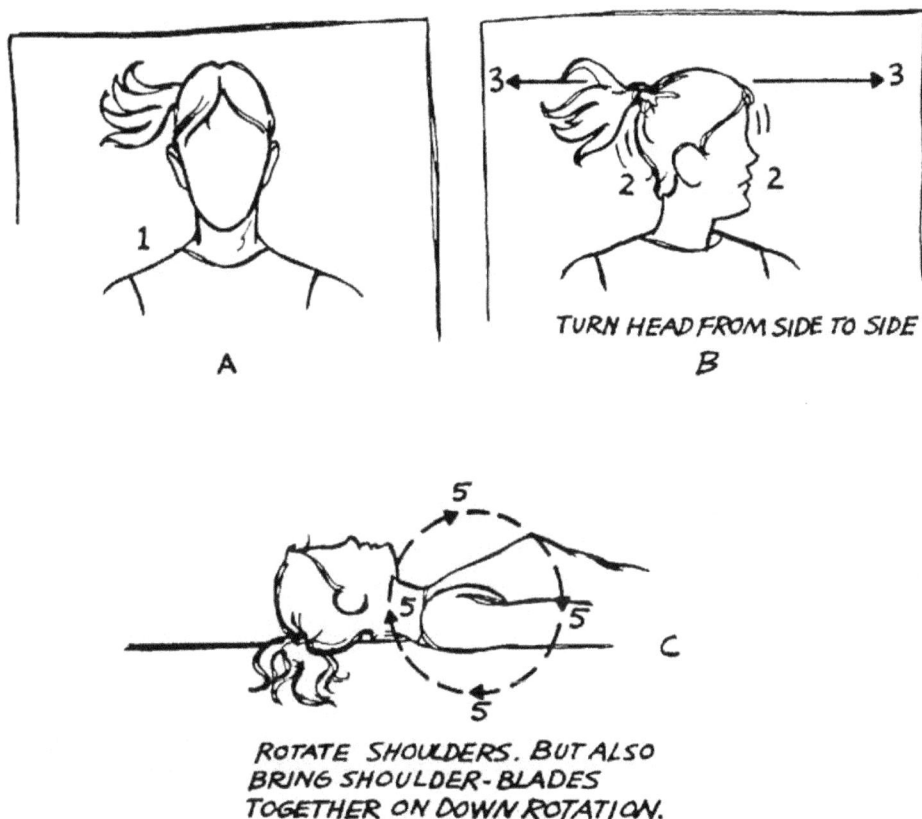

TURN HEAD FROM SIDE TO SIDE
B

ROTATE SHOULDERS. BUT ALSO
BRING SHOULDER-BLADES
TOGETHER ON DOWN ROTATION.

Figure 5
Your Circadian Shock Nullifier

The position to assume (Figure 5A)

1. Lie flat on your back on your bed, with arms and legs comfortably outstretched. No pillow, but no hard surface under your head, either.

How to do this Yoga mov-asana (Figure 5B)

1. Turn your head gently from side to side, first to your right, then to your left.

2. Turn your head all the way to each side, but don't strain your neck. *Continue with* (Figure 5C).

3. Then let your head rest, and

4. Rotate your shoulders footwards, backwards, headwards, and frontwards. After 5-8 repetitions,

5. Rotate your shoulders in the reverse direction, that is, frontwards, headwards, backwards, and footwards. 5-8 repetitions.

Frequency: 3 sets (groups of repetitions). 5 times a week.

What Your Circadian Shock Nullifier does for you:

1. Relaxes your upper back, shoulders, and neck. (A number of important nerve plexuses pass through this region, stimulating the circulation of your brain, eyes, mucous membranes of your nose, thyroids, heart, lungs, diaphragm.) Such relaxation removes the "circadian shocks" from your different circadian rhythms, and restores you to your natural, best-balanced self.

How Ella J. Turned Dynamic Swiftly

At certain times during the day Ella C. suddenly felt fatigued and out-of-sorts. Her work became a nightmare, and to associate with people grew difficult. To stand, sit, or talk pleasantly seemed impossible. The alteration threatened her efficiency, disturbed her relationship with others, and imperilled her chances for romance. But she was afraid to take "pep" pills.

I taught Ella Her Circadian Shock Nullifier. Since she could not find a convenient place where she could lie down at work, she sat briefly in the washroom and did the Yoga mov-asana sitting down. To do it she kept her neck straight, but let it roll from side to side. She also rotated her shoulders. The simple movement was not quite as satisfactory as when done lying down, but it nullified her circadian shocks enough to convert her into a dynamic person swiftly.

Stretching Back Muscles and Spine with a Board

Psychic allergy causes your sympathetic nervous system to respond a bit too fast or excitably to situations. The resulting alteration in you is so minute that it defies diagnosis and passes for normal. But all your "aggression" muscles, from your skeletal to your visceral, are then a little too ready to tense. This state may be erroneously called "nervous tension.'' Relieve your psychic allergy by calming your sympathetic nervous system through feeding your mind with the response of deep muscle relaxation. The Myotatic Relaxer is the Yoga mov-asana for it. Here is how to do it. (Follow Figure 6.)

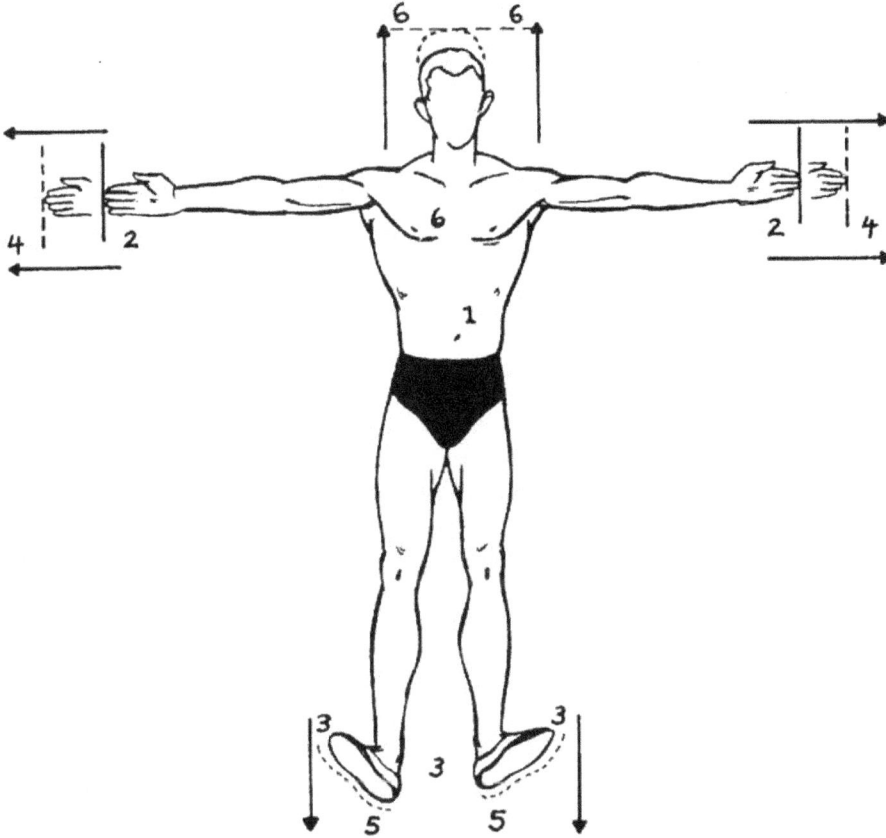

Figure 6
The Myotatic Relaxer

The position to assume (Figure 6)

1. Lie on the floor, flat on your back.

2. Stretch your arms out at your shoulders, like a cross,

3. Have your legs about one foot apart at the heels, and your toes pointing headwards.

4. Now, stretch your arms out sideways *hard*, as if to widen your shoulders. At the same time,

5. Stretch your legs downwards, as if to sever them from your very straight hip joints. Keep your toes pointing headwards! Immediately afterwards,

6. Stretch your back and your neck headwards, as if you are trying to grow taller.

7. Relax and repeat seven times. But stretch sideways, downwards, and headwards farther and farther in each repetition, *all at the same time*, as if to increase your width and height by an inch or two.

8. Each time you relax, relax from head to foot.

Frequency: 5 times every morning.

What The Myotatic Relaxer does for you:

1. Stretches your body effectively and relieves the weight of your vertebrae from your spinal discs. Stimulates you from head to foot.

2. Releases the appropriate alpha wave from your brain, your *own* brain wave of peace and contentment. Stimulates your whole nervous system.

3. By doing this mov-asana lying down, rather than standing up, it stretches your back easier than when done standing, combatting the downward pull of gravity. Stimulates your whole circulation.

4. Restores most of your lost natural height by stretching and straightening your spine. Tones up most of your muscles.

5. Helps to relieve your psychic allergy headache which may have been erroneously attributed to "nervous tension."

6. Helps to slenderize your waist and flatten your abdomen.

7. Makes you taller and broader shouldered. Expands your chest. Triggers your bowels. Improves your sight. Keens your ears, shapes your mind.

8. If you are a woman, it gives you a streamline, wasp-waisted figure.

How Elmer Y. Burst with Joy at 55

Elmer Y. had suffered from an inferiority complex all his life because he was not tall or broad-shouldered enough. From early boyhood he had been bullied, insulted, and mistreated. Every bit of extra height and shoulder-width, he said, added to his protection. But now, at 55, he was even losing whatever he possessed of those assets, and it filled him with anguish. More young people, too, were growing taller and broader!

I taught Elmer the Yoga mov-asana to stretch his back muscles and spine with a board. A week later, he raved, never in his life had he engaged in anything more relaxing. He felt taller and wider-shouldered already, his "nervous tension" headache was relieved, his waist was slenderizing fast, and his abdomen was flattening.

In a month's time he was satisfied that he had *definitely* increased his height and his shoulder-width. His spine and shoulders felt limber, too —ready to lengthen or widen considerably more with this mov-asana. In three months Elmer claimed to have broadened *one full inch* on each side! (At 17 I myself broadened four inches in three months.) He brimmed with joy and, with his new personality, increased his business commissions amazingly.

Yoga Made Safe for Moderns

The Yoga mov-asanas are scientifically designed to protect and strengthen your back. The Yogis, with their limited knowledge of the anatomy of the bones, joints, and muscles, unwittingly injured themselves with many of their strenuous asanas (postures). My extensive background in medical, dental, chiropractic, and body-building knowledge was especially helpful in perfecting the Yoga secrets and in converting them into mov-asanas (moving postures) and bringing you their best possible gains.

All the Yoga mov-asanas which involve your back permit you to arch it backwards *only* when you are sitting or standing, and by jutting your hips backwards *at the same time*. Your lower back muscles always contract then (the erector muscles which hold your back straight) and *limit* the range of the arching to a normal, healthy, muscle-contracting bend. NONE of the mov-asanas permit you to arch your back like an acrobat would when standing, sitting, or lying down, and risk cursing you with a permanent weak sway-back, or even with a "slipped disc."

That's why none of the Yoga mov-asanas (like the YOGAMETRICS simple movements in my book, *Yoga for Men Only*)[2] let you bend your back backwards when it is *loose. That* is why you need the protection of scientific knowledge and application. Different Yoga mov-asanas also build up different portions of your chest (or breasts); trim different portions of your waist; and make powerful (or *glamorize*, if you are a woman) your shoulders, arms, back, and legs. They also avoid frown-forming posture strains, traumatic ligament stretching, questionable hip-joint contortions, debilitating fasts, and other doubtful bypaths of Yoga. But they also tie-in your physical health and body development with your utmost mind-power development and convert you, all at one time, into a mental and psychic giant of health and longevity.

How to Spare Your Spine Throughout the Day
and Escape Back Trouble

There are patients who complain regularly of chronic low back pain. Yet, X-rays and other tests reveal no pathology or curable defect in their spines. Even bedrest or surgery fails to help them. This was described in detail in my book, *Yoga For Men Only*, as far back as 1969. The perplexed physician will exhaust every means of diagnosis and relief, and still fail to relieve the pain. Such a patient is accused of playing a "pain game" on his doctor.

I insist, though, that unless these patients are true malingerers, they are badly misunderstood. You yourself might not suffer from arthritis, but a sudden or prolonged strain could subject you to similar pains. If you are a housewife, you might strain your back from bad posture when washing the dishes, bending over a table, doing the laundry, or ironing. Your sink, kitchen table, ironing board, or laundry machine may be the wrong height for you and regularly compel you either to bend down too low, or to bend back too far and to maintain this uncomfortable position for a prolonged period. The awkward position overstretches or overtenses certain tendons of your back muscles, while it overslackens others.

Or you might strain your back when sitting in an overstuffed or modern chair or couch which curves your back like the letter C and overstretches the muscles and tendons at the base of your spine. When driving your car you have to sit leaning backwards, with your weight thrust upon your lower back, straining its muscles and ligaments. When you walk you might habitually bend too far forward or carry one shoulder lower than the other. You might lean your neck too much to one side, carry one shoulder more forward than the other, throw one foot farther outwards than the other when you step forward with it, and thereby jerk that side of your body abnormally at every other step. You might slump abnormally while sitting, sit twisted to one side when writing in long hand, or let your shoulders "hang" awkwardly and overcompress the vertebrae of your neck.

You might sit or walk too straight and lean backwards habitually on your lower back, or carry a briefcase, handbag, or other "heavy" object too frequently in the same hand, or too long with one hand before changing it to the other. You might stand with a decided sag to your back, lift furniture, jerk windows open or hoist other massive or resisting weights with your knees straight and your body bent forward, instead of with your *knees* bent and your back *straight*.

How to Save Your Spine All the Time

You expose your back to these traumas most of your waking hours. Your back can't endure them without altering over a period of time. Your spine is not a steel beam, but a structure of bone, cartilage, and fiber which changes and weakens over the years when steadily abused. It eventually degenerates into a worn-down, misshapen, arthritic (joints-ruined) relic of a once healthy mechanism and demoralizes you with mysterious pains. It partially incapacitates you far beyond your years.

You can end or greatly reduce such ruinous trauma habits on your back! Do The Myotatic Relaxer (page 27), on several occasions a day to restraighten your spine as much as possible when it is misshapen. And do The Yoga Back Curl, (page 19), to keep your spine normally straight with your sacrospinalis (spinal erector) muscles. Sit down when you don't have to stand, and lie down when you are weary and don't have to sit. Rest your spine from the merciless downpull of gravity and relieve your spinal nerves from the compression of the vertebrae above and below. You will be astonished at how much you will spare your back throughout the day and help insure your living to a ripe old age with a "young" back.

References

[1]Brad Steiger, *Psychic Chicago* (Garden City, N.Y.: Doubleday Doran, 1976).

[2]Frank Rudolph Young, *Yoga For Men Only* (West.Nyack, N.Y.: Parker Publishing Co., Inc., 1969).

2

How Yoga Makes Your Limbs Youthful and Supple for Extraordinary Well-Being

How Youthfully Attractive Limbs Depend on Muscle Tone

When you stop exercising your arms and legs, they lose muscle tone and their appearances suffer. Their skins adapt to the change, and, if you are thin, hug the shrunken muscles and wrinkle. If you are not thin, your arms and legs form fatty lumps which disfigure them. If you are a woman, the fatty lumps show up markedly when you are in a bathing suit or wear short sleeves, skirts, or shorts. If you are a man, they are less noticeable. Your thighs, though, shrink at the knees and bulge more at the hips, distorting your figure. None of these changes adds a youthful look to you. A youthful look requires muscle tone.

How Strength in Arms and Legs Helps You Resist Disease

When your arms and legs are strong, you are inclined to be physically active. Physical activity stimulates your sympathetic nervous system, the system that fights off disease. When you stop being physically active on a regular basis, your body's defenses weaken. To "feel" strong, too, which you do when your arms and legs feel solid, fills you with a positive attitude against disease. You feel confident that you can fight it off, for you feel confident that you can climb three flights of stairs easily, sprint the length of your block, drive your car for long hours at a stretch (which, of course, I don't recommend), play golf over a long course, defend yourself against an assailant, and perform many other physical feats which you would not dream of with soft arms and legs.

When you don't feel well, besides, you can still remain active if your limbs are solid. When you are confined to bed, you recover faster because you can get up and move about sooner. As I describe in *Somo-Psychic Power: Using Its Miracle Forces for a Fabulous New Life,* the tone of your muscles tones your mind, and, reflexly, makes it stronger.[1] With a strong mind you resist disease more easily.

The Miracle Yoga Mov-asana to Strengthen Arms

You feel like a much lesser person than you are when your arms are flabby. Even when you make sound plans in business or in anything else, whenever you face the reality of putting them into effective action, your "wishy-washy" arm muscles won't tune up your mind with the feeling of being a conqueror, and you give in and fail. Your life is ruined by such arms. Overcome this handicap quickly with The Arm Herculizer (which you do more gently if you are a woman). This is how to do it. (Follow Figure 7.)

The position to assume (Figure 7A)

1. Jam a table against the wall, or you can use a sink.

2. Stand before it, with your feet about hip-width apart.

3. Place your palms against the edge of it, each palm about 3 inches beyond the width of your body.

4. Keep your knees practically straight (but not stiff and straight).

How to do this Yoga mov-asana (Figures 7B,C)

5. Bend over far forward, keeping your hips *close* to the sink.

6. Resist your body's bending over by pushing your palms hard against the edge of the table or sink. Wear gloves to protect your palms.

7. As your elbows bend, *try* to keep them perpendicular to the sink. You won't be able to, but prevent them from bending backwards more than halfway (or more than a 45 degree angle).

8. Bend your body over until your arms are fully bent, contracting your biceps fully (Figure 7C).

9. Your palms will then be bent back from your wrists, as well as turned outwards, causing your biceps to contract to a super-peak.

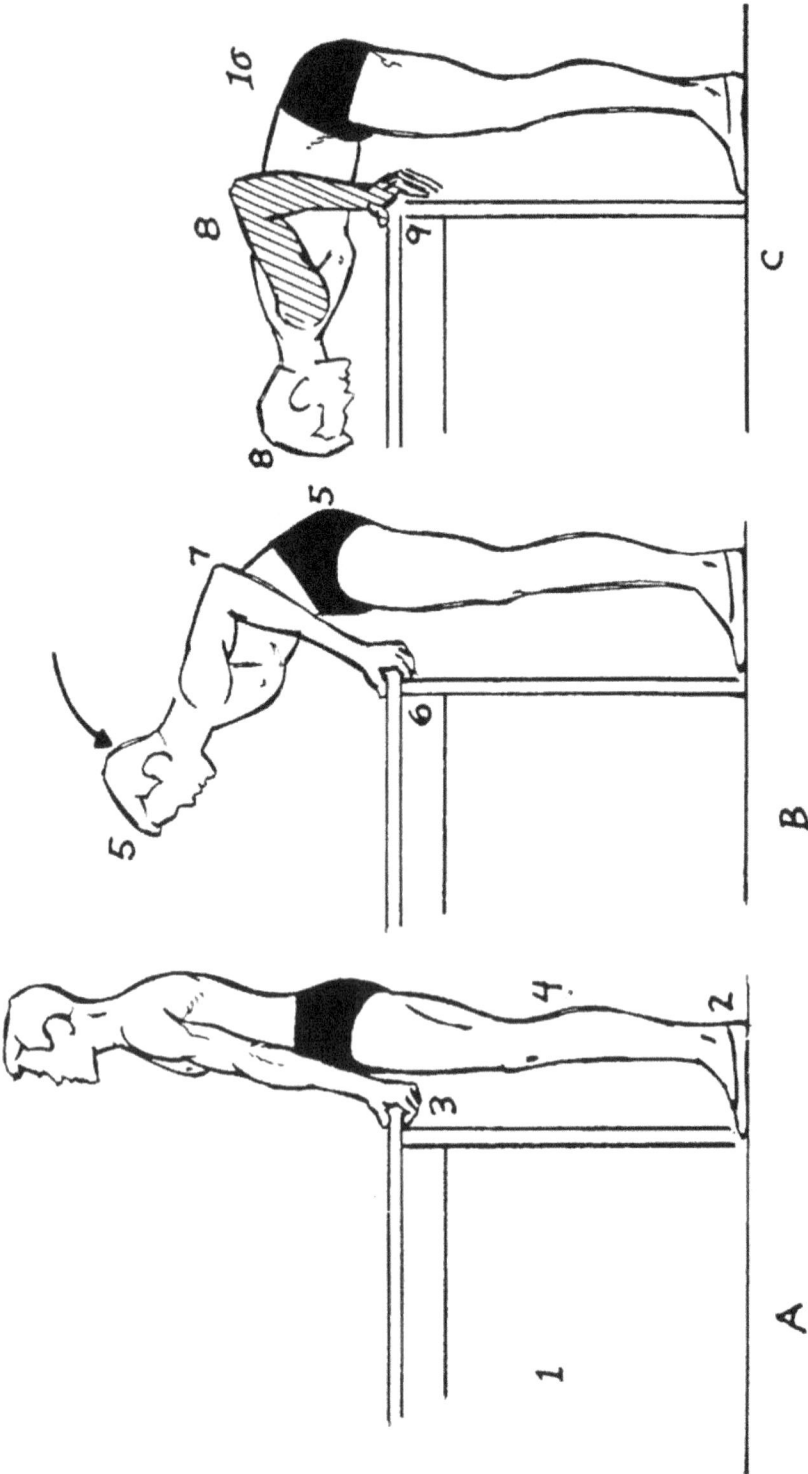

Figure 7
The Arm Herculizer

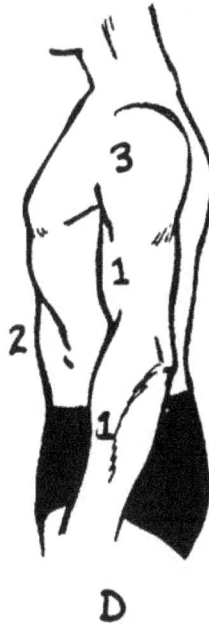

D

Figure 7, cont.

10. The eye-catching muscle of your inner forearm (your brachoradialis, Figure 7D-1) will stand out prominently and build shapely, powerful-looking forearms.

11. Your abdominal muscles will contract hard as you bend over (Not numbered.)

Frequency: 5-10 repetitions. 3 sets (groups of repetitions). 4 times a week.

Note: If you are a woman and don't seek big biceps, do this Yoga mov-asana with half your strength to shape your arms and keep them young, firm, and trim.

What The Arm Herculizer mov-asana does for you (Figure 7D)

1. Gives you large, powerful biceps and forearms.

2. Flattens your waist.

3. Builds up enormously the fronts of your shoulders (your anterior deltoids). Fills you with an invincible frame of mind.

Carl's arms grew quickly with this Yoga mov-asana, and he suddenly felt powerful. His confidence in himself increased by leaps and bounds. He stopped feeling inferior to others when they were merely bigger or held better positions than he. He no longer cowered easily, and stood his ground and defended his ideas. Other people gave in to him, for a change, and his dreams started coming true.

How Earl N. Developed Huge Biceps Fast

Earl N. was 51, but he still harbored the youthful ambition to possess massive arms and a boyish waist. His wife called him childish, but Earl resented observing physically-developed youngsters with giant arms and tiny waists, while his own were flabby and shapeless.

I agreed with Earl that when a man had big, strong arms and a flat waist, his ego received a dynamic impetus that multiplied his chances of success at anything. So I taught him The Arm Herculizer.

The very next day Earl's biceps felt "very sore." No other exercise, he exclaimed in amazement, had "pumped up" his arm muscles so hard. And yet, it required no hoisting of heavy weights; no stretching of dangerous spring or rubber equipment that could snap off and blind him; no swallowing of hazardous steroid- or hormone-exciting pills; no circulation-jamming, extremely painful isometric contractions.

In a month Earl's arms enlarged an unbelievable 1½ inches, and his waist shrank by 2 inches. In ten weeks he possessed big, powerful arms, and the waist of a youth. As a bonus, his chest had bulked up an additional 2½ inches in girth. His wife could hardly believe her eyes.

The Yoga Mov-asana for Shapely Thighs and Shoulders

Your hips, thighs, and shoulders are the foundations of your body. When your hips and thighs are strained, you can barely walk. When your shoulders are strained, you can hardly hold a job or do anything much in your home. The enforced inactivity piles up fat on your waistline; your whole body softens and leaves you prone to still more strains and injuries. Your recreation is limited, leaving you little to live for. The pains and discomforts of these parts of your body are those of arthritis and bursitis. When they lose their shape your whole body loses its proportions. The Yoga mov-asana to keep these parts strong and healthy and finely proportioned is The Torso Push. Here is how to do it. (Follow Figure 8.)

The position to assume (Figure 8A)

1. Stand before something strong and low enough, like your kitchen sink. (Your washroom might not leave you enough space between the wall and the sink for this simple movement.)

2. Don a pair of gloves to protect your palms from the friction. And wear old shoes or pumps that won't slide.

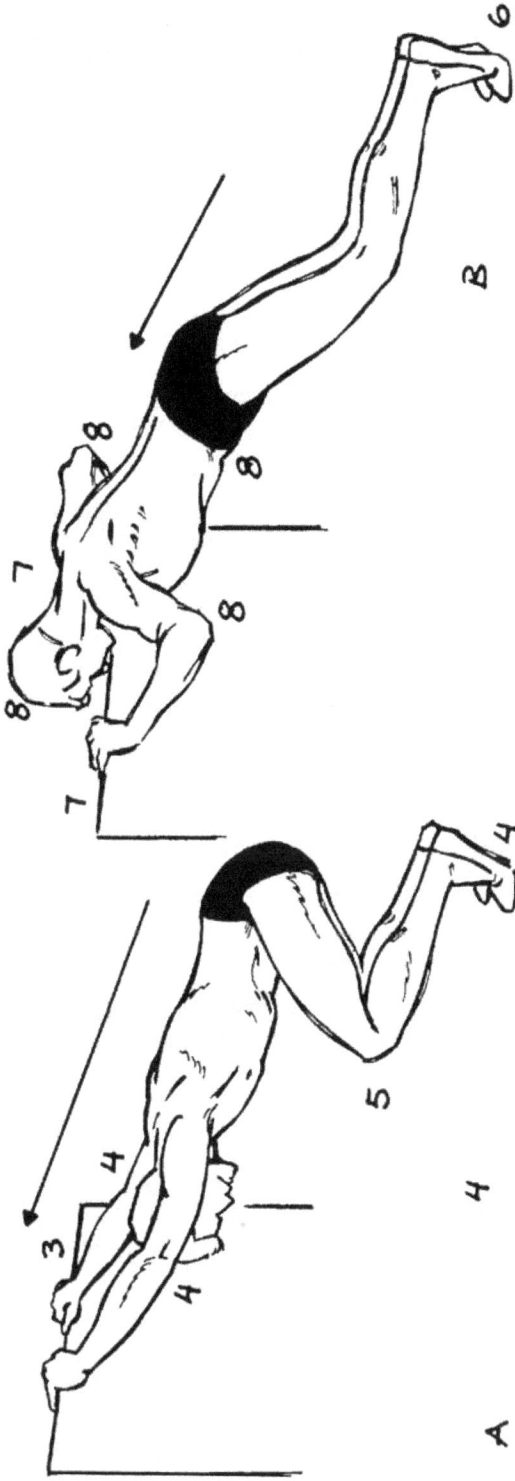

Figure 8
The Torso Push

3. Cup your hands over the edge of the sink, between 2 and 2½ feet apart, depending on your height.

4. Stand back about 4½ to 5 feet from the sink, or far enough to straighten your arms. Have your feet pointing straight before you, about 6-7 inches apart, so that they feel comfortable.

5. Crouch low on your knees, so that your arms are nearly straight.

How to do this Yoga mov-asana (Figure 8B)

6. With balls of feet, push torso upwards at an angle towards the sink.

7. Resist the push with your arms and shoulders. Resist so strongly that your thighs push hard to overcome the resistance. (Don't push nor resist that hard if you are a woman. But push hard enough off the balls of your feet to make your arms and shoulders firm to overcome the resistance.)

8. Keep body crouched low enough, meanwhile, to barely clear the sink with your face as you move upwards. Your arms bend as they give in from the push of your legs.

9. Crouch low again on your knees and repeat.

Frequency: If you are a man, 3-4 repetitions, with strong resistance from your arms. 2 sets (groups of repetitions). 3 times a week.

If you are a woman, 5-6 repetitions, with mild or moderate resistance from your arms. 2 sets (groups of repetitions). 3 times a week.

What The Torso Push mov-asana does for you (Figure 8C)

1. If you are a man, develops powerful, big-muscled thighs. If you are a woman, proportions them in a beautiful, sexy way. Wears off their ugly lumps, firms their skin and smooths them out. If knees get sore, skip 1 week.

2. Draws more blood to your thighs and hips, throwing you into a parasym-

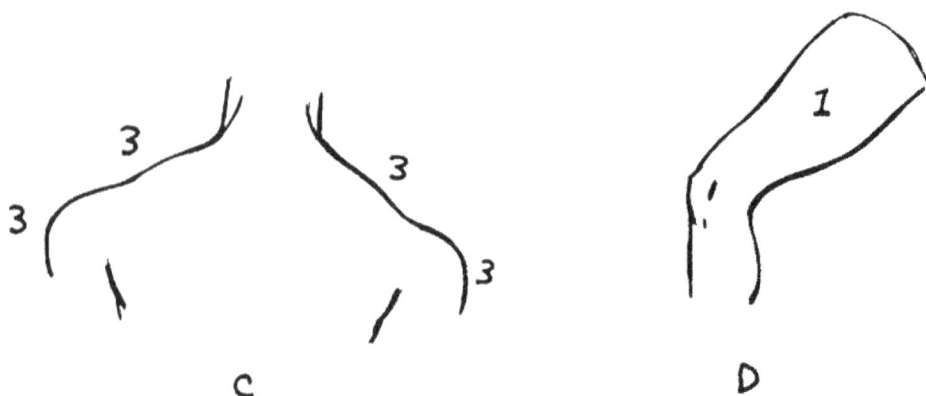

Figure 8, cont.

pathetic nervous system circadian rhythm. You feel gleeful, as a result, and sexually renewed. Turns you romantic; also aggressive in a career.

3. Proportions your shoulders girlishly, if you are a woman. Bulks up the corners of your shoulders into statuesque globes if you are a man.

4. To an extent, helps overcome simple constipation.

5. Strengthens your hip and knee joints.

How Lucius I. and His Wife Used Yoga to Remold Themselves

Lucius I. and his wife, Ethel, were in their 50's. Their children were grown up and graduated from college. Their home was paid for. They had sound investments and money in the bank. Both worked still and were well-paid. But they were dissatisfied with their figures. Their thighs had softened and fattened, and their shoulders were "looking old." When vacationing in sunny places or wearing summer clothing they felt "ancient."

I taught Lucius The Torso Push mov-asana. In a week he and Ethel were aware that their thighs and shoulders were shaping attractively, appearing more youthful. The simple movement drew blood to their thighs and hips, too, and they felt more daring and sexually renewed. It also strengthened their weakening hip and knee joints, the plague of advancing years. With the passing weeks it wore off the unflattering lumps from Ethel's thighs, but carved striking muscles on Lucius'. It blessed Ethel with the girlish shoulders of a young woman, but broadened and filled out Lucius' shoulders. So thrilled were they with their individual changes that they begged to be taught all the other Yoga mov-asanas.

Building Youthfully Graceful Arms with the Easy Yoga Tort

If you want arms that are primarily youthful and graceful, do the Easy Yoga Tort. Whether you are a man or a woman, it will mold your arms into lines most becoming to your sex. This is how to do it. (See Figure 9.)

The position to assume (Figure 9A)

1. Sit comfortably on a stool or on a narrow, armless chair.

2. Let your arms hang by your sides, palms forwards.

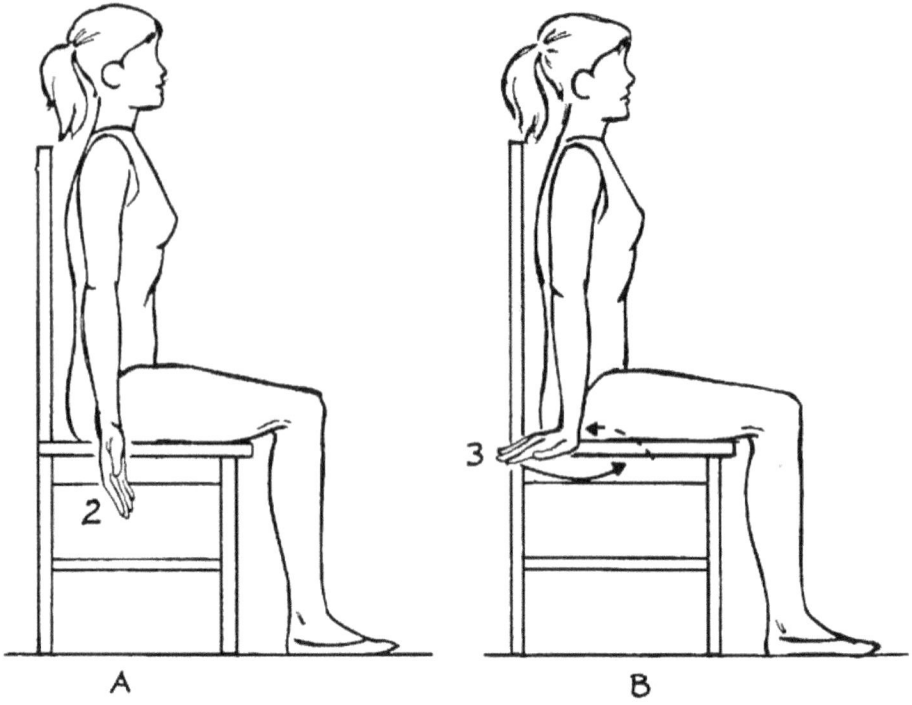

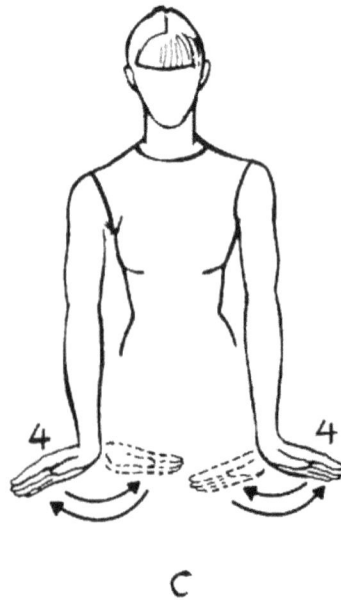

Figure 9
The Easy Yoga Tort

How to do this Yoga mov-asana (Figures 9B,C)

3. Bend your hands upwards to the back of you, palms down, fingers nearly straight. Now,

4. Keep your elbows straight and rotate your hands forward, and then to the inside, so that your fingers point toward your body. Then,

5. Rotate them back to the starting position.

Frequency: 5-10 repetitions. 3 sets. 3 times a week. Do the movement fast.

What The Easy Yoga Tort does for you (Figures 9D,E,F)

1. Firms your whole arm (Figure 9E), but

2. Does not enlarge it because it hardly contracts any of its muscles hard (Figure 9E). Stimulates you with a youthful feeling.

3. Wears ugly fat off your arm because you do it fast (Figure D).

4. But if your arm is too thin, it fills it out nicely (Figure F).

5. If you let your fingers curl instead of holding them straight, your arms will slenderize still more because the muscles will firm less (Figure 9E). But if your arm is too thin or shapeless, then hold your fingers straight and its muscles will fill out more (Figure 9F). Reflexly, speeds up your thinking.

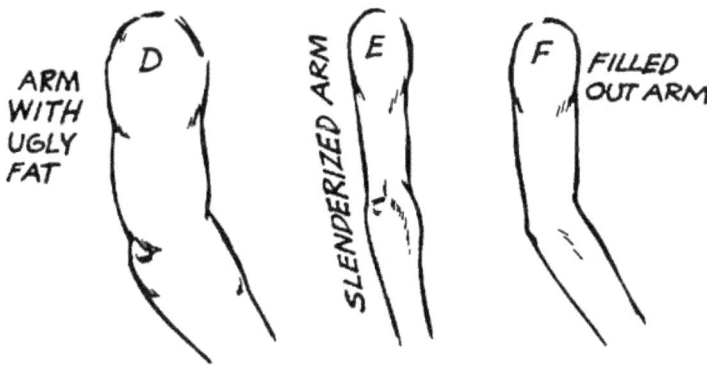

Figure 9, cont.

How Esther W. Thrilled Others with Her Every Gesture

Esther W. was a passably attractive woman, but she had grown ashamed of her arms. Over the years they lost their shape and spoiled her body language. In business she had to deal directly with people and lost somewhat to the younger women whose arms were still attractive because of their youth. Reflexly, too, they had slowed down her thinking.

I taught Esther the Easy Yoga Tort. I was pleased because she did it with vim. Within a few weeks the whole contour of her arms changed. The flabbiness, the shapelessness, the lack of exciting curves, the unflattering disproportions her arms had acquired almost vanished, as if by magic. Her arms soon looked as they did when she was 15 years younger, and led people into accepting her as being considerably younger than she was. Esther's effectiveness in her position zoomed. Her brain sped.

That wasn't all. The bachelor she had kept company with for three years stopped trying to urge her into a "trial marriage," and really married her!

Shaping Your Upper Calves Through a Yoga Mov-asana

Your whole life is a struggle to regain the attractions Nature endowed you with, as well as to try to add new ones. Yet, man and Nature are continually draining you of them. You won't regain the backbone of your attractions unless you strengthen your anti-gravity muscles. Otherwise, you will gradually feel older than you are, and suffer from bad posture, particularly when you stand up or walk. The Yoga mov-asana to regain the backbone of your attractions is Your Upper Calf Shaper. This is how to do it. (Follow Figure 10.)

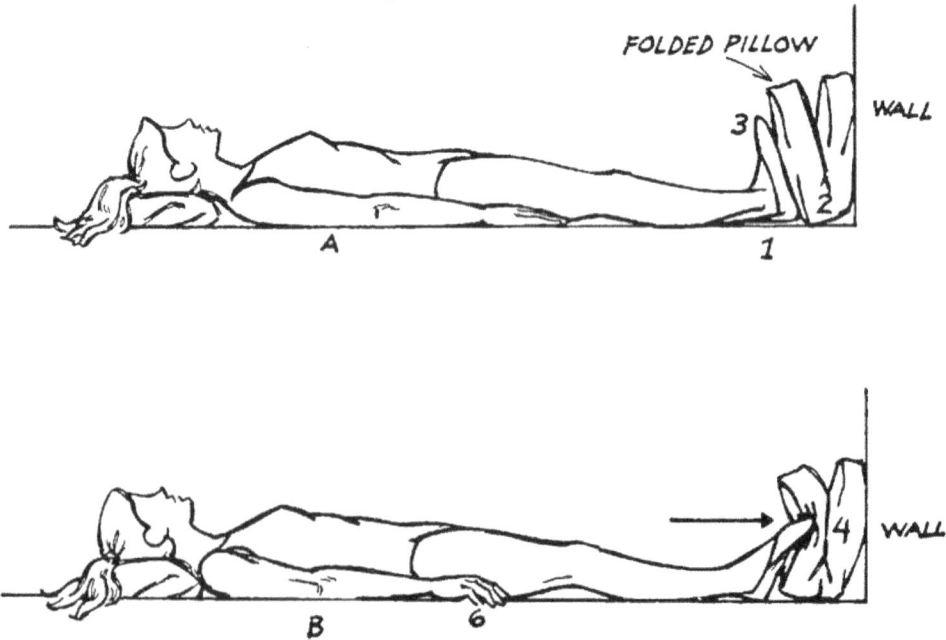

Figure 10
Your Upper Calf Shaper

The position to assume (Figure 10A)

1. Lie flat on your back on your bed, or on the floor if it is soft enough. Place your feet close to the bedstead, or to the wall if you are on the floor.

2. Fold a pillow to keep it thick and resistant, and place it between your feet and the bedstead or the wall.

3. Point toes headwards, and sink heels deep in pillow.

How to do this Yoga mov-asana (Figure 10B)

4. Press with the balls of your feet—*pigeon-toed*—deep into the pillow, as if to push the jammed pillow into the bedstead or the wall.

5. Repeat.

6. Hold onto the sides of the bed, if necessary, to prevent your body from being shoved away from the pillow. If you can't hang onto something (particularly if you are on the floor), wiggle back to the pillow after every two or three repetitions.

Frequency: 10-12 repetitions. 2 sets (groups of repetitions). 3 times a week. 5 times a week if your legs need more shape.

Do it one day with your feet pigeon-toed (or turned inwards). Next day, with your toes pointing upwards. The third day, with your toes pointing outwards.

What Your Upper Calf Shaper mov-asana does for you:

1. Glamorizes every contour of your calves.

2. Erases the knock-kneed look, the bow-legged look, the spindle-leg look, the thick-ankled look, the knotty-calf look. Adds grace to your moves.

3. Strengthens the anti-gravity muscles of your calves and makes unavoidable long standing, walking, or other leg strains easier to endure.

4. Lessens the possibilities of developing varicose veins or broken capillaries in your legs and thighs by strengthening the muscles that support those blood vessels. And,

5. Since it is done lying down, it relieves those blood vessels of your weight, instead of straining them all the more, as when you stand and use weights or work, and risk developing varicose veins. Fills you with optimism.

How to Have Strong Bones All Your Life

Regularly eat foods like beans which contain a high percentage of calcium. Sun. yourself regularly, too, or try to spend at least one hour a day outdoors to absorb vitamin D-triggering sunshine. Even if clouds and man-made pollution prevent a large percentage of the sun's rays from reaching you, enough of them will to enable your body to absorb the calcium from what you eat. Otherwise, your bones will turn porous prematurely as you grow older.

To *retain* the calcium in your bones, eat the least amount of refined foods, such as white sugar and white bread, as possible. These extract too much calcium from your bones. Eat moderately, also, of prunes, tomatoes, rhubarb, cranberries, and spinach. These contain too much oxalic acid. The same applies to cereal and grain. The latter contain too much phytic acid. Both acids combine with the calcium in your bones and excrete it in the form of insoluble salts. A quantity of these salts also remain in your kidneys and can eventually accumulate and form kidney stones.

Exercise regularly, too. The healthy strain on your bones from resisting the scientifically-designed Yoga mov-asanas promotes their regrowth and their hunger for calcium. Since your natural glandular changes due to age cause your bones to retain less calcium as you grow older and turn more porous and brittle, do Yoga mov-asanas all year round. The healthy strain also causes your bones to produce more action current electricity in your body and to fill it—and your mind—with daring energy.

References

[1]Frank Rudolph Young, *Somo-Psychic Power: Using Its Miracle Forces for a Fabulous New Life* (West Nyack, N.Y.: Parker Publishing Co., Inc., 1974).

3

How Yoga Produces a Body
That Is
Youthful, Slim, and Appealing

Ways Yoga Banishes Overweight Conditions

The Yogis are masters at maintaining their normal weights. Their diets are stringent, but the Yogis also hold to a dictum that everything in Nature tends to balance itself, and that your body tends naturally to stabilize its own weight. My medical great-grandfather propounded the same principle a century ago. I myself have repeated it since my college days.

To reduce beneath your normal weight is practically impossible —unless you put yourself under unnatural influences, such as taking appetite-ridding drugs, engaging in dubious or dangerous fasts, having sections of your intestines removed, subjecting yourself to near-scalding steam baths, undergoing kidney-imperilling dehydration (such as by abstaining from drinking water for days at a time), eating far less food than normal, and so forth. The Yogis contend that some part of your brain controls your body's efficiency in processing your food. In other words, when you become heavier than your "ideal" weight, your body automatically loses weight to regain its efficiency. While, when you become lighter than your "ideal" weight, your brain demands more food to restore you to your "ideal" weight to regain your lost efficiency. Your organs, your bones, your muscles, and your other tissues, after all, possess a normal weight for their size. Your brain instinctively knows what that weight is, and it regularly strives to keep your body normal by maintaining these organs at their normal sizes.

Eliminating High-Calorie Foods the Easy Yoga Way

The Yogis, as far back as is known, have favored peanut as a protein. Famed nutritionists agree with them now as to its unusual value. Dr. Tze Chiang of the Engineering Experiment Station of the Georgia Institute of Technology in Atlanta reports that peanut flour has about ten times the mineral content of wheat flour, five times as much as protein, and is much richer in vitamins. Several food companies, as a result, are producing peanut meal by crushing peanuts. So, peanuts should not be condemned as being "fattening." (Keep away, though, from salted peanuts.)

But you don't have to starve yourself to slim down. Eat three meals a day, with a full breakfast and supper. Also have a filling lunch, but one which is easily digested. But consume enough bulk with each meal to prevent yourself from over-eating fattening foods. Add some protein to it, like eggs, meat, fowl, fish, or peanuts at breakfast and supper. Although I don't recommend oils if you find them hard to digest, you may add a few drops of corn oil, safflower oil, soybean oil, peanut oil, or olive oil to your vegetable bowl at breakfast and supper. Like the Yogis, however, I find that practically all oils noticeably retard digestion. There is enough oil in the foods themselves which contain them, foods like peanuts and soybeans.

I doubt, though, whether oils when eaten, smooth out the skin, as much as is believed. Mainly, they add submucous fat to the skin, which helps to camouflage the actual wrinkles. But, at the same time, they add ugly fatty lumps around the waist and thighs, particularly if you are a woman. (Wheat germ oil, of course, in large quantities, can also reduce your weight. But it can also disturb your hormone balance.) About five peanuts or three walnuts a day should provide your body and your skin with all the oil you require and not overburden your liver.

How Yoga Lore Helps You Choose Natural Foods

Yogis, of course, consume no artificially-condensed foods, nor take vitamin or hormone pills. They don't "juice" their foods and flood themselves with juices. Dr. Basil Brown, a 48 year old Ph. D. in chemistry in England, drank up to a gallon of carrot juice a day. He died of vitamin A poisoning. It brought on a state similar to the cirrhosis of the liver caused by alcoholism. When he died, his skin was bright yellow from five years of that diet. Dr. Brown had suffered from health problems and was convinced that large doses of vitamin A would improve his condition.

An accumulation of vitamin A can cause you to lose your appetite. It can cause sparseness of hair, liver enlargement, and yellow skin diseases. The same is true of vitamin C. Despite the wide publicity it has received, I myself find that large doses irritated the bladder and urethra. Other researchers[1] found that instead of protecting against colds, they even *decreased* the body's vitamin C content. And a top medical researcher[2] found that they also increased the chances of heart attack by elevating blood cholesterol. It is wiser to eat a sensible diet and, like the Yogis, neither eat nor drink anything to extreme.

Avoid seasoning your foods and let your taste glands select for you the foods to eat. Your body knows best what it needs more of, and it flashes that command to your taste glands. Don't prevent your taste glands from doing their job effectively by seasoning your food and deluding them into accepting *the seasoning* as your whole food. Season the *worthy food* then, not the worthless food. But it is better to season *none* of your food and let your appetite remain normal and select for you only what your body chemistry commands it to. Seasoning, besides, leads to overeating because you enjoy the seasoning more than the food.

Let the foods themselves season each other, in fact. Let the juice in the carrots and beets sweeten your salad. If the salad is too dry, add some natural juice to it, or even a natural oil if you can digest it easily. Some tomato juice or a helping of beans is even better.

Particularly, don't season the meat and other foods which you should eat sparingly. Eat the least of foods with exceptionally good taste, such as desserts, ice cream, fancy bakery goods, and so forth. Give your taste glands a fair chance to protect you from disease and loss of health! With his taste glands the cat avoids harmful foods and discovers healing herbs when he is ill. Let yours protect you likewise. You won't have to build up your willpower at the table then, and can enjoy eating and still take care of your health without even trying. The Yogi lets his own Nature guide him and reaps the rewards by living a long, healthy, active life.

How Yoga Eliminates the Need for Fad Diets

As far back as 1954, in *Solar Diet*, I urgently recommended three square meals a day. "NEVER try to skip breakfast," I wrote. I also insisted that "your breakfast has to be big enough to fill your stomach to the point where it will stimulate your intestines to contract (peristaltic wave) so that your bowels feel like emptying. A small breakfast will not usually do this." (*Solar Diet*, p. 16) "To reduce," I continued on pages 56 and 59, "You can't afford to starve yourself, either. . . you *still* have to put bulky, healthy food into your system, or [you will] starve yourself and turn constipated. . . The same principles apply for losing weight. When you eat too little, you not only feel weak, but you also bring on constipation.'' About 20 years later (1974), science has found those conclusions to be true, practically word-for-word.[3]

Regularly trying to ''keep slim'' can afflict you with a condition known as *anorexia nervosa*, or a compulsive self-starvation. You would soon be extremely weak and suffer from disorders of your glands and hormones, stomach ailments, serious mental disorders, and even end up in suicide. Perpetually watching your weight, besides, turns you self-centered, and you can think of nothing but yourself. If you are attending school or college at any age, you will be unable to absorb yourself fully in your studies or achieve anything else worthwhile because your dieting weakens you or absorbs your interest abnormally.

The Value of Slight Excess Weight Around the Waist

Slight excess weight around your midsection, anyhow, is *natural*. Abdominal flesh adds fat naturally, even when a specimen of it is grafted onto the arm or leg. Slight excess abdominal flesh supports your abdominal organs like a truss, and in addition, keeps them warm. But you need *no more* than four extra pounds of it. Don't shrink yourself to the degree when your abdomen looks ''lean.'' To maintain that look requires regular dehydration (or abstinence from drinking water). Several prominent old-time prizefighters dehydrated themselves to ''make weight'' for lucrative contests with lighter men. Many succumbed later to pneumonia or kidney disease. Others, like Gene Tunney, lost one kidney 25 years later. Many body-builders dehydrate themselves for as long as three days prior to contests like Mr. America or Mr. Universe, in order to appear at their trimmest—and risk, in time, permanent health damage.

Trimming down too fine, besides, robs your skin of beautifying subcutaneous fat and encourages it to wrinkle early and deeply. This is all the more true if you are over 30. Many a 50-ish woman who reduces 15 pounds or more to be healthier and look younger, looks 15 years older, instead. Loose skin then hangs under her arms, forms ugly rings around her neck when she moves, and furrows her face. Eating too little, also, may constipate you because it deprives your bowels of its necessary stimulating bulk, and brings on hemorrhoids, appendicitis, and, eventually, possibly diverticulitis (pockets of trapped waste matter in your colon), and cancer of your lower colon and rectum, probably due to the trauma of trying to move hard bowels across their mucous membranes.

The Safe Way to "Manage" Your Weight

To control your weight safely, then, eat a well-balanced diet, with fruit and cereal (unprocessed) roughage added to your breakfast, and a good helping of fruit at lunchtime. Eat a normal supper, with lean or organ meat or fish. Exercise sufficiently four to five days a week to wear off your excess body weight without trimming yourself down into an early wrinkling, kidney-disease threatened state. Every day spend a few minutes doing at least 3 sets of 2 of the mov-asanas listed under Slimming and Reducing (in Index) to draw in your waistline from the front and sides without fasting or dieting. Within a varying period of time, depending upon how overweight you are, you will reach your ideal weight. And you will be satisfied with your meals and look the least wrinkled for your age. If your excess weight is pathological, of course, see your doctor or healer. (When your weight increases from 5 to 10 percent without a significant change in your eating, exercising, or other contributing living habits, it is considered pathological.)

Ending Your Fear of Calories

The Yogis don't know what calories are and don't fear them in the least. You don't have to fear them, either. Not all food calories fatten you, anyway, and some calories are vital to your good health. Some Yogis fast before deep psychic absorption. For health, though, they don't. They learned, thousands of years ago in their vigorous lives, that a starvation diet decreased both the energy requirements and the energy expenditures of their bodies. The Yogi also found out that he could gorge himself on energy-creating foods, and yet not fatten. An experiment at the Oak Knoll Navy Hospital in Oakland, California, upholds this.[4] It was found that a low carbohydrate diet (but with sufficient protein and vegetable oils), caused volunteers to lose a total of 13 pounds, but less than one-half pound of lean tissue. (Lean tissue is the muscle, liver, blood cells, etc., in your body.)

Many researchers have upheld the findings. When you are reducing, then, add other calories which cause reduction of your body fat (through oxidation) but restore and maintain your lean mass. You will waste away, otherwise, and look and feel old and be more susceptible to disease. You have to add a certain amount of protein and fat-containing calories to your food in order to rebuild and maintain your lean tissues. The polyunsaturated fats (vegetable oils) are far less fattening than the saturated animal fats. Carbohydrates, or sugars and starches, however, cause fat production and fat storage in you, just like the saturated animal fats. So, to control your weight, greatly curtail such foods as the Yogis do.

What the Yogis Do About Calories

The Yogis go still further. They don't take vegetable oils. They depend upon the natural food itself, and, in addition, upon bulky food to remove fat like that being absorbed in the alimentary tract. Their stomachs would find the concentrated vegetable oils heavy and slow to digest. Without realizing the scientific reason why, then, the Yogis rely upon bulky food to remove the excess fat in their foods and avoid burdening their digestions with concentrated vegetable oils.

Lastly, you utilize your food more efficiently early in the day. Yet, Americans eat almost 80 percent of their food after 6 P.M. So, to lose weight, eat a big breakfast, as Harry D. did. (His story follows.) It is not so much how much protein you eat, but *when* you eat it. If you eat it early in the day, you will derive more benefit from *less* food—and lose weight without fasting.

How a Western Student of Yoga Shed 40 Pounds Effortlessly

Harry D. had tried many different ways to reduce and was deeply disappointed. He was 40 pounds overweight, and worried deeply about it. It ruined his figure and alarmed him about his future health. He did lose weight with the different methods he tried, but they left him weak and flabby and so badly starved that the moment he discontinued them he "ate like a horse" and fattened up all over again.

I revealed to Harry the scientific Yoga secrets to reduce and stay reduced—without starving himself. So, he ate two heaping vegetable bowls a day, one at breakfast and one at supper. Each contained several leaves of lettuce, a grated small carrot, a grated small beet, one shredded stalk of celery, a quarter of a cucumber, and a small portion of some other vegetable in season, like green pepper, radishes, zuccini, or any other kind. To add more taste to the bowl at breakfast, he added two small apples or pears, or some other fruit in season. Watermelon was one of his favorites because it filled him as well, and stimulated bowel movement. A small helping of fish supplied the necessary protein.

At breakfast Harry also ate five prunes, half a handful of raisins, four walnuts, grated to save his teeth from the trauma of chewing them, and two glasses of skim milk. Had he been among those who have been told they cannot digest milk (a conclusion to which I still don't subscribe heartily) he could have substituted an unsweetened fruit juice like pineapple for the milk.

This bulk-containing breakfast, plus the glass of warm water which he drank upon arising, helped by His Appetite Controller mov-asana, promoted a massive, weight-reducing bowel-movement in Harry. Although his breakfast contained a satisfactory quantity of needed calories for health and strength, the mass of food bulk in it combined with, and removed from his intestines, a vast quantity of food fat.

For supper Harry added sliced tomato or tomato juice and cooked dried beans or lentils to his vegetable bowl. He also consumed a small portion of fish, liver, lean meat, or the like. Also, one slice of bread (not white) with a thin covering of natural peanut butter, and finished with two glasses of skim milk (or unsweetened fruit juice, if he preferred).

For lunch Harry ate two bananas (or three whenever he chose), and drank a glass of orange juice.

Between meals he drank only water whenever he felt thirsty or hungry. Once a week he added some ice cream or pie to his supper.

How the Western Student of Yoga Grew Stronger as He Lost Weight

Harry walked and jogged for 15 minutes, three times a week. He took nothing to reduce his appetite at meal time. Indeed, I urged him to eat all he wanted—particularly of the vegetables. The more food-bulk you consume the more fat it carries out of your body. So Harry felt neither hungry nor weak between meals. Indeed, he felt pleasantly full and strong. He drank more water in the afternoon because his lunch filled him less than his breakfast or supper. But it also compelled his body to use up its extra weight to supply his muscles with needed calories for his daily activity. He did the Yoga mov-asanas he liked best and developed a remarkable shape as he lost weight. His chest, back, and shoulders grew hard with muscle, while his waist slimmed down to that of a youth.

Harry felt so much stronger and solid that he was hardly aware that he was reducing. He lost just so much weight, for he was not starving himself. He ate no candy, mixed no sugar in anything he ate or drank, avoided cholesterol-forming cream and other fancy dairy and bakery products. He skipped carbonated drinks, beer, candies, chocolates, and unnecessary desserts. He not only lost weight but transformed himself into a powerful, much better built, far more energetic person. Yet, he ate his fill of the foods listed. As he lost weight, he added from five to ten dried dates to his lunch. In fact, I advised him to add some to it from the very beginning if he felt that he needed more calories for the afternoon.

I didn't want Harry to lose weight in crash-diet style, but in a gradual but positive manner. I wanted him to retain his full strength (actually, he increased it immensely!), and not acquire a thin, drawn, old-looking face and old-looking, hanging body skin. I wanted him to look—and feel —much younger, not older.

People who had not seen Harry for months could hardly recognize him. He had lost nearly 30 pounds. He was "wearing off" the remaining 12 in the same manner, and looking—and feeling—younger every day. Harry turned much more handsome and acquired admirable proportions.

A Yogi's Torso-Trimming Secrets

A Yogi's efforts to achieve union with the Absolute requires the

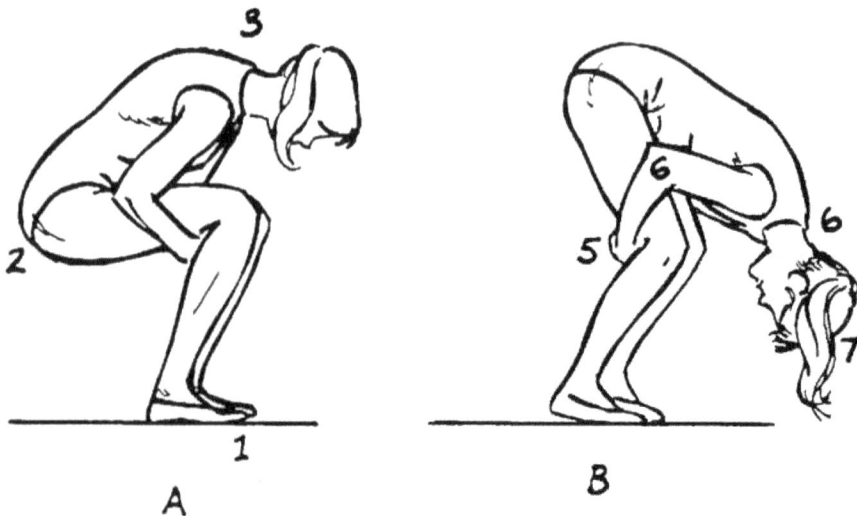

Figure 11
Your Appetite Controller

clearest thinking mind to draw out his Hidden Powers in a flash. Such a mind has to be helped by a torso which won't waste energy-carrying blood by locking it up in capillaries lost in masses of fatty tissue. The Yogi, for that reason, makes sure that his torso is always trim. Your Appetite Controller is the most effective mov-asana to achieve that end. Here it is. (Follow Figure 11.)

The position to assume (Figure 11A)

1. Stand with heels hip-width apart.
2. Squat way down to your haunches.
3. Bend body forward as much as possible.
4. Hug your bent-over body tight to your thighs.

How to do this Yoga mov-asana (Figure 11B)

5. Straighten your knees, but

6. Still hug your thighs and keep your body bent forward as much as possible.

7. Squat way down again and repeat. It is a very simple movement.

Frequency: 2 repetitions. 2 sets (groups of repetitions). 5 times a week.

What Your Appetite Controller mov-asana does for you:

1. Flattens amazingly the front of your waist (Figure 11D). ·
2. Brings blood to your head to flush your brain with oxygen, its food.

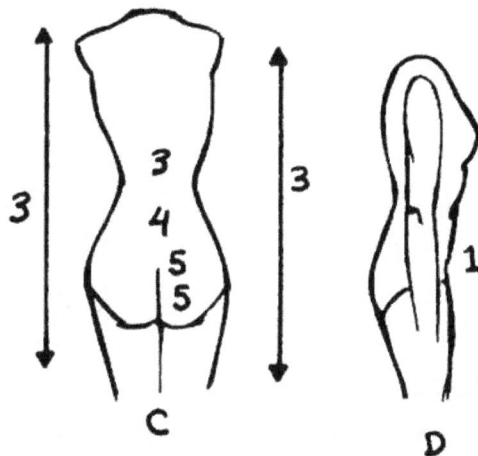

Figure 11, cont.

3. Stretches the "kinks" out of your back—particularly your lower back—much like traction therapy (Figure 11C-3). You will feel the effects of this thrilling stretch after you stand up at the end of a set. (If you suffer from back trouble, of course, seek professional help.)

4. This back stretch helps relieve arthritis of your lower back (Figure 11C-4). I know cases in which the condition no longer bothered the sufferer, and he felt as if he were cured. Fills your brain with nerve-electricity.

5. Stimulates your sacrum and coccyx (the bones at the back of your hips, at the base of your spine), thus improving your bladder, legs, and sciatic conditions (Figure 11C-5).

How Charlotte F. Easily Controlled Her Weight

Charlotte F. enjoyed nibbling at her food all day long. She didn't overeat at the table, but her total food consumption was more than she suspected. She was alarmingly overweight and was convinced that she could never control it.

I taught Charlotte Her Appetite Controller mov-asana. It "shrank" her stomach (or drew in her waist) to the degree where she did not feel hungry for hours after a meal. I advised her to limit herself to three meals a day and to drink a glass of water whenever she felt hungry between meals.

It was soon no problem for her to control her appetite between meals. Her stomach, as a result, "shrank" still more. In a few weeks her weight was down to normal, and her waist was remarkably small. And yet, she had stopped watching her diet and ate practically anything she wanted to. I also advised her, though, to select her food with more care. Charlotte controlled her weight easily thereafter and stopped watching her diet "like a hawk."

The Secret Yoga Food That Electrifies Your Tissues

Your natural powers to combat disease vary from time to time. Doctors prescribe medicine primarily to control the symptoms of a disease, not to "cure" the malady. A medicine powerful enough to kill germs inside you would kill your tissues first. But when the debilitating symptoms of a disease are controlled, your body's defenses can resist that disease at their strongest.

The Russians, like the Yogis, use a "secret" food which electrifies your tissues into superb immunity to a great many diseases. The food is garlic. Its oil is sold in Russia in a pill form called alliacin. Garlic is used in Russia for respiratory diseases, like colds, sore throat, bronchitis, pleurisy, and tuberculosis. It is used to lower blood pressure, to eject worms, and for practically every illness for which antibiotics are used in the West. When taken regularly with meals (as described in how to heal sore throat, page 94) at least twice a week, it protects you against influenza and some other communicable diseases. It is said to cure venereal disease by attacking the infectious bacteria in your urinary tract when the sulphur and iodine in the garlic pass through it in your urine. It does likewise to kidney infections. You are warned, naturally, against the dangers of self-diagnosis and self-medication.

But you ought to eat garlic at least once or twice a week with heavy meals. It will electrify your tissues by stimulating your sympathetic nervous system (your ''fighting'' nervous system) and thereby increase your body's natural defences against disease. Within an hour or two after you eat the garlic, you will burst with energy, even if only for a few hours at first. When you take it with your second meal that week, you will be recharged with energy (nerve-electricity) even longer.

The Yoga Mov-asana That Practically Vanishes Your Midsection

The Abdominal Knee-Chest Curl practically vanishes your midsection because it shortens the muscles of the front of your abdomen and draws it in flat. Here is how to do it. (Follow Figure 12.)

The position to assume (Figure 12A)

1. Lie flat on your back, with your
2. Hands holding onto the sides of the bed.
3. Legs straight down.
4. Inhale.

How to do this Yoga mov-asana (Figure 12B)

5. Exhale. At the same time
6. Bend your knees and
7. Draw them up, *pressed tightly together*, to your chest.
REMEMBER: Keep both knees *tightly together*.
8. Raise your upper body off the bed as high as possible, to help bring your chest and knees together.

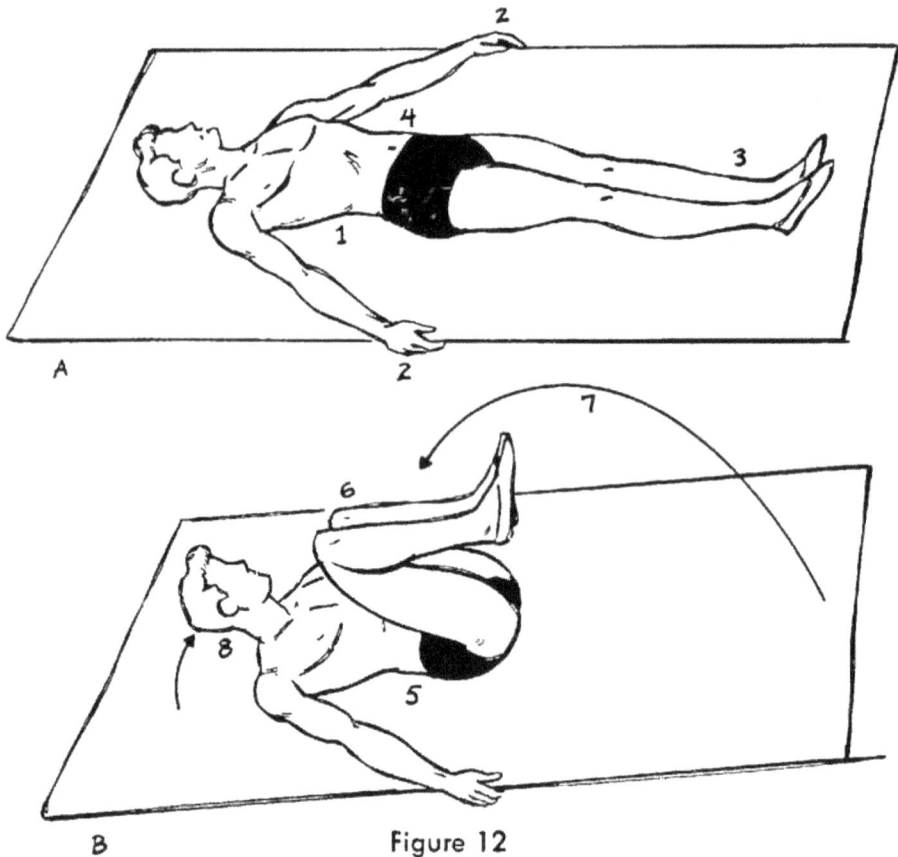

Figure 12
The Abdominal Knee-Chest Curl

What the Abdominal Knee-Chest Curl mov-asana does for you:

9. Quickly wears off the fat on the front of your waist.

10. Is a tremendous aid to uncomplicated constipation if done immediately upon arising in the morning and accompanied by drinking from two to four glasses of water.

Frequency: As many as you like. To wear off your abdominal fat fast, a total of 50 or more every morning, pausing a few seconds in between, now and then, to rest. It is a very simple movement.

How Zella E. Quickly Slimmed Her Waist

Middle-aged Zella E. had a "nice" figure, in general, and was universally admired for it. She could pass for being ten to 15 years younger than she was. But a padding of fat on the front of her waist made her abdomen look "like a tub," she cried with mortification. Try as she might, she couldn't get it off, and she suffered from constipation, as well.

I taught Zella the Abdominal Knee-Chest Curl mov-asana. She did it in the mornings after arising and taking three glasses of warm water, one after the other. It had a magical effect on her bowels and ended her uncomplicated constipation. With the passing days it also wore off the fat from the front of her waist. The sensational figure which Zella pined for was soon hers. So many men—many half her age—tried to date her after that, and so many of them proposed to her, that she had to display her wedding ring *prominently*. But even that was of little avail. The mov-asana had made her *too beautiful* now, she sighed.

The Healthiest, Most Easily-Digested Between-Meals Drink

The average American thinks that he has to drink coffee between meals when he is thirsty. Other Americans and nationalities prefer tea, beer, soft drinks, fruit juices, vegetable juices, light wine, or processed preparations, like Ovaltine. Few are satisfied with plain water; and of these, many will touch only distilled or spring water. Ordinary tap water, they insist, is dangerous because it contains chlorine, minerals, or even sewage.

Yet, ordinary tap water is the healthiest, cheapest, and most easily-digested between-meals drink. (In undeveloped parts of the country and in certain foreign lands, of course, you have to boil the tap water first for about 20 minutes, as a precautionary measure). Common tap water contains no alcohol, tannic acid, or the chemical compounds found in beer, wine, tea or alcohol. Neither does it require digestion, which beer, fruit, and vegetable juices and processed preparations do. Being neither acidic nor alkaline, it does not disturb the healthy milieu of the stomach. (But read on for more on water.)

The Health Magic of the Cheapest Natural Drink

Non-filtered tap water is actually better than distilled water because it usually contains minerals like calcium (hard water). Calcium is a leading food for your heart, for the walls of your arteries (to prevent hemorrhaging), and for your nerves and bones. The chlorine in tap water, besides, is in suspension form. It rises out of the water, like air bubbles, when you let the water stand in the glass for awhile. But the chlorine happens to destroy vitamin E. So boil the water first, if you wish, for three minutes, to force off the added chlorine and neutralize the resulting chlorine compounds. If it is also contaminated with dangerous factory wastes, of course, procure bottled water.

Water, finally, adds moisture to your skin and helps it retain its youthful look. It dilutes and lessens the concentration of wastes in your blood. It flushes the wastes out of your kidneys and bladder. Water cools your body, softens your bowels, and reduces constipation. It fills your stomach enough between meals to discourage an unwholesome appetite for snacks, smoking, alcoholic beverages, enamel-wearing gum-chewing, candy-sucking, and the like. By "purifying" your blood it also keeps your brain clearer. Water is the Number One and *only* liquid which the Yogi habitually imbibes between meals, for it won't dilute your gastric juices and impede the thoroughness of your digestion. Too much of it during or soon after a meal balloons your stomach. Don't drink it at a meal, nor before one and one-quarter hours after a meal, or it will flood too much potassium out of your body. (Your heart-muscle needs potassium.) Then drink about one glass of water every hour until an hour before your next meal. Upon arising in the morning, drink one or one and one-half glasses of warm water, for a total of six to eight glasses a day, all between meals. In cold weather drink less, unless you are thirsty. In warm weather drink more.

Don't worry if drinking water drives you more frequently to urinate. Water is a natural diuretic and will cleanse your blood, kidneys, and liver. But drink none at or after supper if it will disturb your night's rest with trips to the bathroom. One trip at night won't bother you much, but three trips would indicate that you should not drink at bedtime. If you are a man, the long pressure at night on your prostate while you are asleep with a full bladder might irritate the gland, too.

Generally tap water is helpful, however; the amount of tap water you drink costs comparatively little, even when it consists of part of your rent. And it will not make you "big and fat." A prominent scientist concluded that "There is no relationship between getting fat and drinking large quantities of water." I myself have imbibed between eight and 12 glasses of water in big cities for three-quarters of my life and have little trouble keeping my weight normal. "Too much" water-drinking can add, at most, about three to four pounds of weight to your body. Boil the water first, as stated before, and let it cool to drive out the chlorine and compounds it might have formed. If you live in an area in which the water is polluted (such as by factory wastes, etc.) drink bottled water.

Your Easy Yoga Hip Trimmer

Many Yoga postures (asanas) stretch the hips and keep them trim. But they usually strain you and take too long to do. Your Easy Hip

Trimmer Yoga mov-asana is equally effective and does not strain you, nor take up much time. It is the quick, easy way to slenderize your hips. This is how to do it. (Follow Figure 13.)

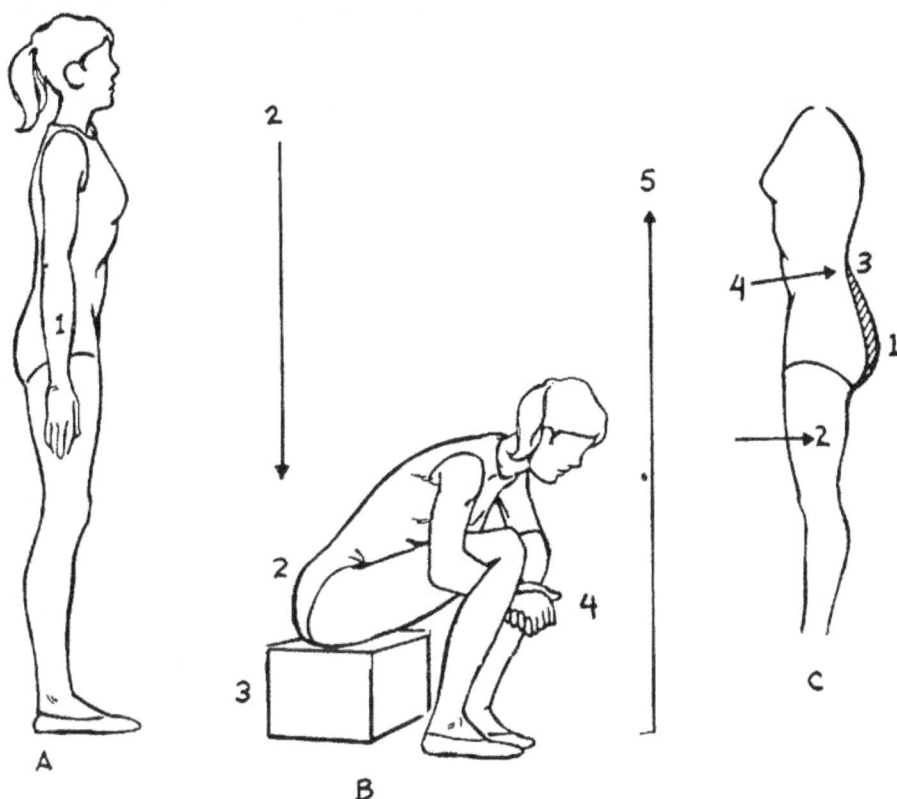

Figure 13
Your Easy Yoga Hip Trimmer

The position to assume. (Figure 13A)

1. Stand straight, with room around you. Let your arms hang loosely by your sides.

How to do this Yoga mov-asana. (Figure 13B)

2. Squat down deep to your haunches.

3. Have a pillow, a thickly folded blanket, or something similar lying behind you to prevent your buttocks from bouncing off the floor, should they drop that low.

4. To maintain your balance as you squat, bend forward and wrap your arms around your calves.

5. Straighten to position No. 1 and repeat.

Frequency: 10-15 repetitions. 2 sets (groups of repetitions). 5 times a week.

What Your Easy Yoga Hip Trimmer does for you (Figure 13C)

1. Stretches your hips to the utmost and wears fat off fast.

2. Shapes your thighs.

3. Wears the fat off your lower back.

4. A fine aid for constipation, especially if done after taking 3 glasses of water. Also relaxes your mind.

How Wanda A. Trimmed Away Her "Bottom Spread"

From adolescénce Wanda A. had been ashamed of her figure. From her waist up, and from below her hips down, her figure was admirable. But her hips were "way too big," as she so accurately expressed it. She had dieted, exercised, taken pills, dehydrating baths, and everything else she had heard of. But nothing had slimmed her hips.

I taught Wanda Her Easy Yoga Hip Trimmer mov-asana. She could hardly believe her eyes at the end of the first week when her hips were already a half-inch thinner. She continued with the mov-asana feverishly in the second week, for it also regulated her bowels. Her thighs, too, were looking impressive! At the end of six weeks she had lost 1½ inches from her hips. Seething with ecstasy, she continued with the simple mov-asana and lost still more. In less than four months she had lost a total of 3 inches in hip girth. Her clothes fit her quite differently, and potential suitors flocked around her. Her mind, too, she said, felt "so relaxed."

How Yoga Lets You Enjoy Eating Again

Your accepted incorrect daily diet may lead to inflammation of your intestines (enteritis) and contribute to kidney infection. Insufficient daily intake of plain water adds further to your misery by permitting the constant presence of certain salts in your urine, like oxalates, which might even cause kidney stone. Your incorrect diet, such as when it contains too much sugar, could even bring on a state in you similar to sugar in the blood in diabetes and irritate your kidneys still further.

It is wise, therefore, to eat balanced meals with plenty of fruits and vegetables. Erroneously called "acid" fruits, pineapples, oranges, and grapefruits actually *alkalize* your stomach and your blood because they are oxidized in your stomach to alkaline. Eat no more than six ounces of meat a day (although many authorities limit it to four ounces). Avoid all tea, coffee, liquors, and artificial stimulants. But drink from six to eight glasses of plain water a day *between meals*. Avoid fatty foods, such as bacon, coconuts, Brazil nuts, ham, and too much pork.

Don't exercise sooner than two and one-half hours after a "digestible" meal. Don't overeat oxalate-containing foods, such as tomatoes, rhubarb, prunes, cranberries, or spinach. Four to five prunes a day are enough. Unless you are under your physician's or healer's instructions, don't "go crazy" trying to find the "right diet," if there is such a thing. I am closely informed about the San Blas Indians and other longevity-famous groups of people in Latin America, like the Andean mountain people. My medical and dental ancestors were associated with them a century and a half before me. These peoples never heard of proteins, carbohydrates, vitamins, enzymes, calories, trace minerals. They live in miasmatic air, heavy with pollution from their coal and wood fires. Yet, many are believed to have lived to 150 and older, and a startling percentage of them are centenarians. But their diets are balanced and have contained no concentrated foods. They do eat coconuts, but they eat them when the coconuts are young, soft, and jelly-like, and not after they have matured and hardened into concentrated fat.

How to Fill out Nicely Your Eye-Catching Neck-Shoulder Lines

From front or back, your neck-shoulder lines are the most striking segments of your appearance. This is true whether you are a man or a woman. Your neck-shoulder line catches the eye of the beholder at once and either draws him to you, or sends him from you. If it is a striking line, it suggests youth, health, dependability, and symmetry. If it is not striking, it suggests that you are older than you are, in bad health, are indecisive, and physically distorted. Perhaps no other achievement in life will reward you more, second-per-second expended on it, than a nicely filled out, eye-catching neck-shoulder line. The secret Yoga mov-asana to acquire it is Your Neck-Shoulder Line Perfecter. Here is how to do it. (Follow Figure 14.)

The position to assume (Figure 14A)

1. Stand before your kitchen sink or anything you can push against with force.

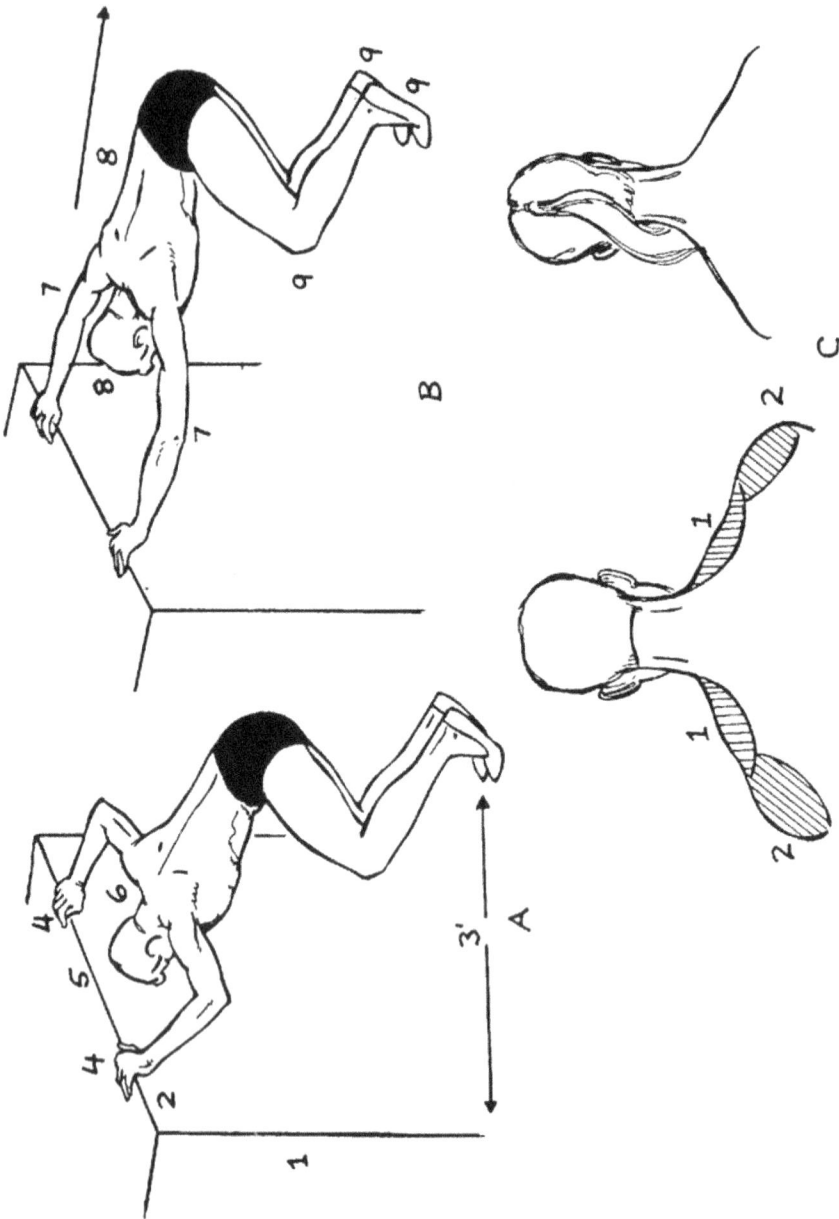

Figure 14
Your Neck-Shoulder Line Perfecter

2. Don an old pair of gloves so you won't feel the hardness of the sink when you push. Also wear a comfortable pair of slippers so your bare feet won't rub against the floor when you resist the push.   '

3. Step back about 5 feet, depending on your height. Now,

4. Lean forward and rest your palms on the edge of the sink.

5. Set your hands about 2½ feet from each other (depending on your height).

How to do this Yoga mov-asana (Figures 14A,B)

6. Drop your body forwards, and place your head *lower* than the level of the edge of the sink. Then

7. Push your body back with your arms until they are fully extended (Figure 14B).

8. Keep your head and back no higher than the edge of the sink.

9. Resist the push by bending your knees and pressing your body forward with the balls of your feet.

Frequency: 3 repetitions. 2 sets (groups of repetitions). 2 times a week.

What Your Neck-Shoulder Line Perfecter does for you (Figure 14C)

1. Fills out the line of your shoulders from your neck outwards. This beauty feature (if you are a woman) will capture the eyes of men when you wear clothes which display your shoulders. If you are a man, it makes you stand out in a crowd and "hypnotizes" everybody you meet.

2. Firms the top of your shoulders so you won't tire easily from sitting or standing and working as the day wears on.

3. You can thereby maintain the different circadian rhythms of your internal systems regularly poised in *effective balance*.

The Secret Potent Concept of Your Neck-Shoulder Line Perfecter

In your normal, everyday life you don't react to experiences in the same way all day long. The changing circadian rhythms of your different organs alter your whole physiology from one hour to another. With your nervous system, though, your neck-shoulder line is a *potent concept*. With it you *can* maintain your different circadian rhythms poised in *effective* balances and remain stable all day long, no matter what you face. Filling out nicely your eye-catching neck-shoulder lines equalizes the muscle tension of both sides of your body by developing them evenly. The two sides of your body then automatically fire all day long to the motor (muscle-commanding) centers of your brain equal "feelings" of power. Your brain, in turn, fires these "feelings" to the glands and viscera on both sides of your body *evenly*, instead of unevenly, as it does when the two sides of your body are not equally toned or developed. Your tendencies to instability are immensely stabilized thereby and your temper and your energy brought automatically under mental control all day.

How Amanda F.'s Figure Suddenly Held Others Spellbound

At certain periods of the day Amanda E. felt so dead tired that she detested her duties. Her shoulders hung like great weights, and she turned grouchy. Whatever natural beauty she possessed left her at such times. As a last resort, she turned to stimulants. But she dreaded acquiring the habit.

I taught Amanda Her Neck-Shoulder Line Perfecter. With the *very first repetition* she felt the shelves of her shoulders firming. During her brief rests between sets her "dragging" shoulders already felt as if being held up by invisible pulleys. The "killing weight" on her arms was gone. By the time she completed the third set, she felt as if she could never get tired again.

A week later she felt practically tireless. Her shoulders no longer "hung down" on her, no matter how actively she worked. Her mind no longer turned grouchy at different periods of the day, nor did her efficiency suffer.

Additionally, as an added bonus, she felt that whatever natural beauty she possessed remained with her all day long, no matter how actively she worked. Indeed, the lines from her shoulders to her neck filled out so enticingly that they captured the eyes of men, particularly when she went out wearing clothes, like evening gowns, which displayed her shoulders. Amanda turned amazingly popular and soon had an enviable list of suitors from which to select a desirable husband.

The Best Least-Time to Exercise Per Week

One of the questions which students of my books and courses repeatedly ask is, "What is the least time to exercise per week to get the most benefits?"

The answer differs for each individual. If you gain weight easily, exercise longer and do more repetitions of each Yoga mov-asana, but make them a little easier. If you are slender and wish to gain more bulk (if you are a man), or more roundness or fullness (if you are a woman), do less repetitions, but resist each one harder and build up your contours instead of trimming them down.

If you are overweight, trim yourself down by exercising five times a week. If you have time, six times a week is preferable. But change every other day to different mov-asanas to prevent your muscles and joints from being overused in the same movements.

If you are underweight, build up your body by exercising as little as three to four times a week. Use full force with each repetition, but rest on the following day to let new tissue build up in you.

Jogging three or four times a week is highly recommended. If you are young enough and engage in competition, jog as much as five times a week. Alternate between two days of distance running and two days of sprinting and walking. To run five days a week after 30 could afflict you, in time, with arthritis of the knees or hips. The over-erect position of running and propelling your legs backwards overarches your lower back like an acrobat's. Such a movement, when repeated for years, could wear down the posterior widths of your spinal discs prematurely and cripple you with arthritis of your lower back.

Note: Jog, preferably, on soft ground or on a running track. The trauma of running on hard pavement can, in time, cause arthritis of your knees. The mov-asanas alone, however, are sufficient for your whole body—and great for your mind, too.

Triggering Your Kundalini for a Striking Chest or Breast

The kundalini has been defined as being "psychic energy—located in the spine." It is the physical source of the miracle power of healing of the Yogi. Make it your own with the Yoga mov-asana, The Brachial Bow. Here is how to do it. (Follow Figure 15.)

The position to assume (Figure 15A)

1. Jam two chairs against a wall, just far enough apart to let you stand between them. (Second choice: a table, bedstead, or a sink.)

2. If you are using two chairs, stand between them. Otherwise, stand close to the furniture selected.

3. Draw arms far backwards, *with elbows hugging sides*.

4. Place hands against the backs of the chairs, elbows slightly bent, fingers pointing downwards.

5. Inhale deeply.

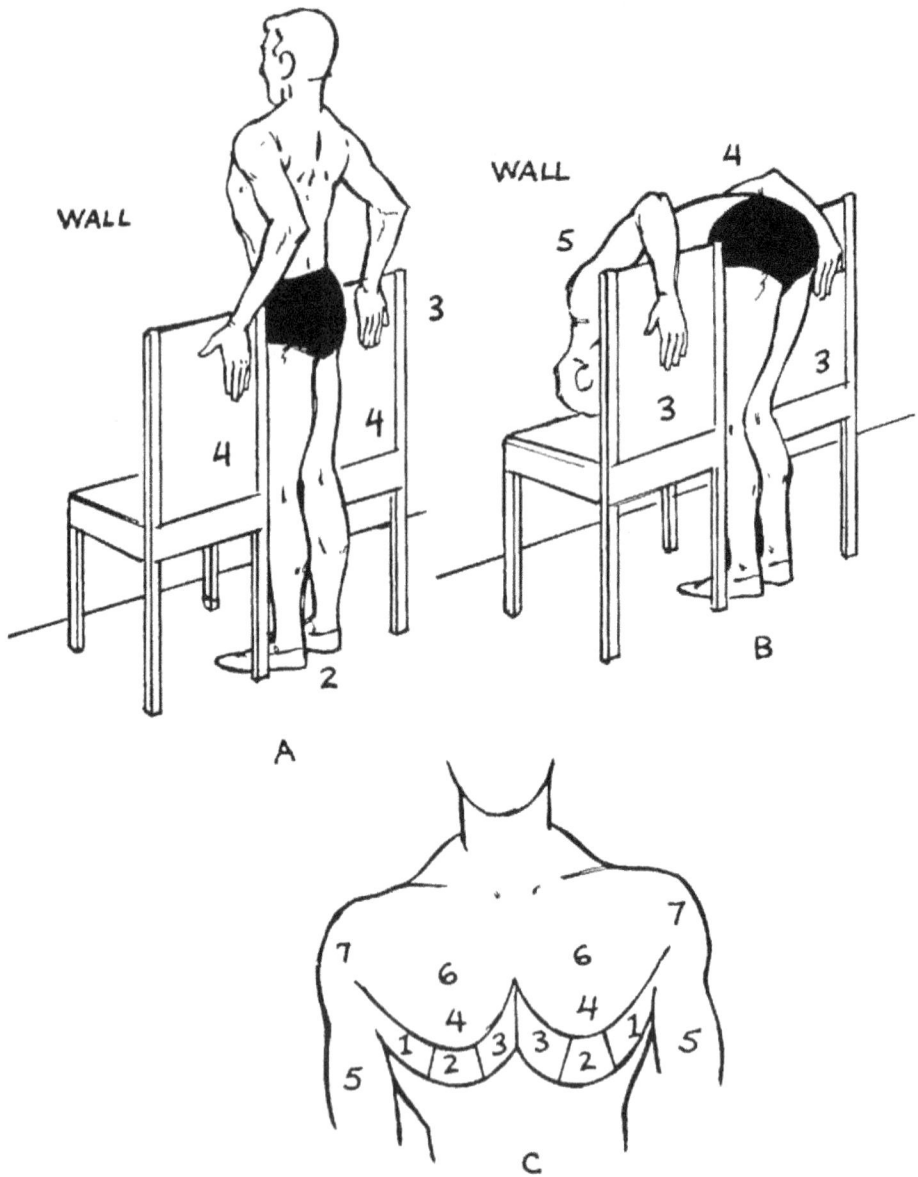

Figure 15
The Brachial Bow

How to do this Yoga mov-asana (Figure 15B)

1. Round your shoulders (Figure 15A).
2. Keep elbows hugging sides (Not numbered).

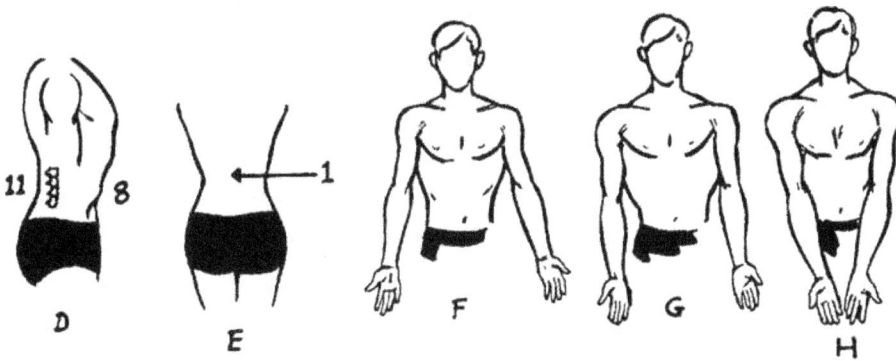

Figure 15, cont.

3. Press all your might with your palms (Figure 15B-2).

4. Resist by locking knees and hips. But *keep them slightly bent* to avoid straining your knee joints. As a result,

5. Your body bends forward and downward.

6. Exhale as your body bends.

Frequency: 3 repetitions. 2 sets (groups of repetitions). 3 times a week.

What the Brachial Bow mov-asana does for you (Figures 15C,D,F)

It proportions you so strikingly that you note the following gains promptly:

1. Wide grip (Figure 15F): the outer borders of your chest muscles (or breasts, if you are a woman) (Figure 15C).

2. Medium grip (Figure 15G): the lower borders of your chest (or breast) (Figure 15C).

3. Close grip (Figure 15H): the lower half of your chest or breast groove (Figure 15C).

4. All three grips fill out the lower middle part of your chest (or breasts) (Figure 15C).

5. All three grips fill out the fronts of your arms (Figure 15C).

6. If you push until your head bend down low, all three grips also fill out your upper chest (or breasts) (Figure 15C).

7. The outer and middle grips proportion the fronts of your shoulders.

8. If you draw your hips inwards, too, and bend both your knees and your body down still lower, this mov-asana flattens your waistline tremendously (Figure 15D).

9. If you are a man and want huge biceps, resist hard with your body as you bend over. If you are a woman and want sylph-like arms, resist moderately with your body.

10. This is an easy, but exceptional Yoga mov-asana. Gives Herculean power and muscular bulk, if you are a man. Gives thrilling symmetry, if you are a woman.

11. Stimulates the vertebrae just above your waist (your 10-12 dorsals), and of your lower back (your 1-4 lumbars) (Figure 19D). Your bladder, uterus, and lower bowel improve. Fills your mind with a feeling of euphoria, which is tremendous for romantic aggression or profitable creativity.

How Oona L.'s Mere Appearance Bewitched Others at a Glance

Oona L. grieved because she was just "one more nobody." She stood out nowhere, was pursued by no one she wanted, and lamented about passing her whole life in obscurity socially, romantically, professionally, and in every other way. She had lost her incentives and felt "down in the dumps."

I taught Oona The Brachial Bow. She found it amazingly easy to do. It remolded her breasts and arms, and her whole symmetry altered into a girlish one. Best of all, the bending over against her arm resistance stimulated the lower vertebrae in her back and triggered the vital energy—the psychic energy in the network of nerves at the base of her spine. This network, her sacral plexus, stored the explosive nerve-electricity of her kundalini.

Whenever Oona completed the sets and walked away, her breasts, arms, and shoulders poured her kundalini power out of her, like the ensnaring aura of a mystic. Thereafter, whenever she met people she liked (and even those she didn't like) and reproduced this feeling, her kundalini power flashed through their bodies and altered their vibrations into rapport with hers. Their bewitched response was immediate! She even made the sick feel better at a glance! Oona's whole life changed. She was soon being pursued by everybody whom she wanted to pursue her.

References

[1]Gerhard N. Schrauzer, chemistry professor at the University of California at San Diego. *Science Digest*, May 1975.

[2]Dr. Leslie M. Klevay, research medical officer at the U.S. Dept. of Agriculture Human Nutrition Laboratory at Grand Forks, South Dakota. *National Enquirer*, Aug. 10, 1975.

[3]David A. Levitsky, a physiological psychologist at Cornell University.

[4]Dr. Hilde Bruch, professor of psychiatry at Baylor College of Medicine in Waco, Texas.

[5]*Science Digest*, July, 1972.

4

How Yoga Helps People of All Ages Develop Healthy, Attractive Skin, Teeth, Gums, Eyes, and Ears

---

A Yoga Method of Preventing Skin Aging (Nine Secrets)

Skin cells themselves, it seems, become more susceptible to cancer as you get older. Simple aging, besides, reduces the amount of elastin fibers in your skin. Your skin no longer stretches out smooth as it did in your early years. You yourself accelerate the process, though, by inflicting unnecessary traumas on your skin. Limit the traumas and you will look, as you advance in years, from 20 to 30 years younger than you are. Here are the Yoga secrets to limit them:

1. Stop wrinkling your face unnecessarily. Stop squinting, for instance. Stop narrowing your eyes when you peer at things. Stop raising your brows and wrinkling your forehead when you speak. Stop wrinkling your nose when you assume different expressions. Stop pursing your lips habitually. Stop walking or sitting with a slumped back and throwing your neck backwards and wrinkling it in the back. Stop frowning when you concentrate. Stop sulking regularly and making your cheeks look sunken and hollow. None of these habits add to your impressiveness. They make your skin look only prematurely old.

2. Stop smoking. Tobacco smoke irritates the whites of your eyes (your conjunctiva) and streaks them with blood-shot veins. Your face muscles, in addition, wrinkle the skin around your eyes in their reflexive efforts to protect your eyes from the smoke, and the wrinkles turn permanent in time. The muscles of your forehead also tighten that skin into frowns, and these also eventually turn permanent. Dangling a cigarette habitually between your lips purses them and also wrinkles them prematurely. Even when you hold a lit pipe or cigarette in your hand, smoke seeps into the air and contracts your facial muscles.

69

3. Don't strain to read fine print unless you consciously relax your eyes and brows or wear reading glasses. Straining your eyes to read contracts the muscles around your eyes and contributes to crow's-feet. The over-concentration to read the difficult print causes you, besides, to frown and look older.

4. Wear glasses when you go out (not corrective glasses, if your eyesight is good enough), to avoid squinting from the wind. They also protect the whites of your eyes from the lacerating traumas of sharp dust particles in the air which cause them to redden. Wear sunglasses to neutralize the blinding sun-ray reflections from windshields or high-rise windows, which can injure your retina so badly as to lead to blindness. (More about this in another Yoga secret.)

5. When you plan to remain outdoors with clothes on, longer than one hour, smooth something protective on your face. A face-protective oil or liquid would do to ward off the trauma of excessive cold or heat on your face and diminish your self-protective wrinkling. But rinse off the application with water of normal temperature when you return home to unplug your pores. When the weather is too windy or icy, better stay home altogether, or your skin muscles will over-wrinkle your face to combat it.

6. Engaging in skiing, boating, and similar outdoor sports regularly subjects your skin to abrasive contact with the wind or sun or both and ages it prematurely. It may be necessary to cover your skin then with protectors or even to apply Vaseline or a similar product.

7. Don't stand often near hot ovens, radiators, furnaces, stoves, or any other high temperature devices. The excessive heat dries out your skin and brings on premature mosaic-type wrinkling.

8. And, of course, don't sunbathe too long at a time. Oil yourself, too, first. Don't lie in one position longer than 15 minutes at a time. If the sun is hot, change your position as often as every five or six minutes. Also, immerse your body in water, or take a shower, or cool your exposed parts by pouring water over them once every hour to cool them, or your skin will turn too hot and dry out. After cooling your skin, also apply more oil to your body, including your face. These precautions are great protections against freckles, ugly areas of pigmentation which could, in time, change into cancer, sunburn, and premature drying out of your skin.

9. Two hours of sunshine at a time, unless the sun is very cool, are sufficient. You need but one hour of sunshine a day to absorb the vitamin D in your food. But you can take another hour for pleasure, such as swimming, bathing, or diving. If you sunbathe longer than one hour at a time, cover your skin thickly with protective oil and keep your skin cool.

Yoga Protection Against Skin Cancer

The rugged outdoor exposures of the Yogis threaten them with skin cancer. They protect themselves against it with regular consumption of yellow fruits and vegetables, such as mangoes, papayas, carrots. Science upholds them now with the recent discovery by Harvard University scientists that beta-carotene protects against sunlight. Beta-carotene is found in yellow and green leafy vegetables and yellow fruits. It enables persons super-sensitive to sunlight to stay outdoors four times as long without developing redness, burning, swelling, and itching. Ingest the beta-carotene in your normal diet because too much of it will give your skin a yellowish color.

How Wrinkles May Be Reduced

Repeatedly during the day, and even when you sleep or dream, your thinking and your volcanic emotions draw your brows tight with muscle tension and stamp them with the "harassed look." Your brows form into noticeable, forbidding "swells" and lend your face an aloof, austere, older aspect. Your physiological (circadian) rhythms function increasingly *out of step* with each other as you grow older, anyway. That's why, as the years march on, you acquire extreme sensitivity to slight changes in schedule, to small doses in drugs, and to moderate changes in light, temperature, or noise acuity. These changes manifest themselves in your emotions and contract the muscles of your scalp, face, neck, and upper body. These emotions regularly form unnecessary wrinkles on these parts and add from five to 15 years to your apparent age. Overcome this natural handicap and look much younger by considerably reducing the wrinkles on these parts of your body. The secret Yoga mov-asana for it is Your Luring Brow. This is how to do it. (Follow Figure 16.)

The position to assume

1. Sit and face your image in the mirror.

2. Visualize your brows as bulging tight beneath your skin (for they are) (Figure 16A).

3. Make yourself aware of that tightness and of the petulant, irritable, harassed, antisocial aspect it lends your face.

How to do this Yoga mov-asana (Figure 16A,B)

4. Stare at the space between your eyes. Imagine that your eyes are so close together simply because your tight brows are drawing them that near. Assume that if you could relax your brows, your eyes would shift wider apart. Now,

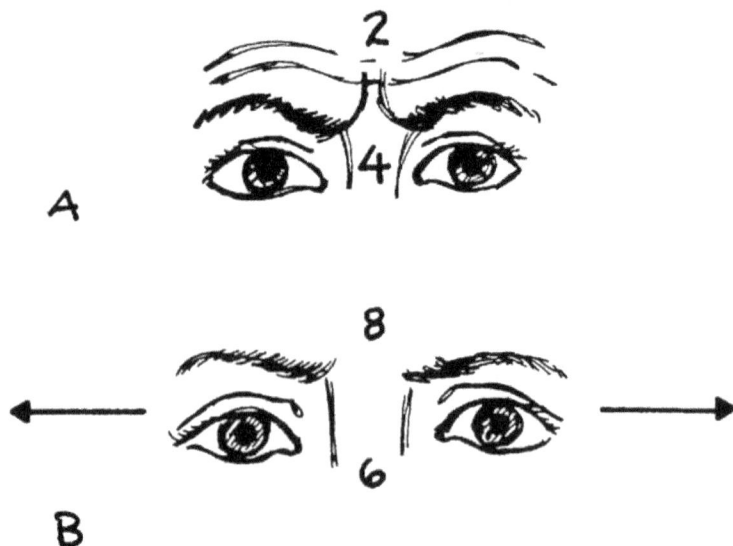

Figure 16
Your Luring Brow

5. Visualize yourself shifting your eyes wider apart with sheer willpower. Stare at the small space between them and ''see'' it widen.

6. Try to follow the direction of the side-shifting of each eye. Your left eye will then look as if it is more to your left, and your right eye as if it is more to your right—*both at the same time* (Figure 16B).

Frequency: 10 times a day. 5 days a week.

The results of Your Luring Brow mov-asana

7. Your external eye muscles relax a little and let your eyes drift farther apart, as they do when you sleep or gaze lazily into space.

8. Your brows follow suit, due to the reflex connections between their nerves and those of the external muscles of your eyes.

9. After a little practice (in a week or less) your brows will relax when you *merely think* that your eyes are wider apart than they actually are.

What Your Luring Brow does for you:

1. Relaxes your scalp, face, neck, and upper body, due to the reflex connections between their nerves and those of your brows. The wrinkles on your brows instantly reduce. When done regularly your expression wrinkles will practically vanish, and new ones will be prevented from forming.

2. Conquers tension headaches produced by the tension of the muscles of your scalp, neck, and upper body.

3. You look much younger in an instant. Your mind turns inventive.

How Cynthia E. Looked 20 Years Younger at a Flash

Cynthia E. was 58, but she craved to look much younger. Hers was a natural and normal wish, but she didn't know how to achieve it. She did not seek plastic surgery, and was opposed to wearing more make-up. Dieting made her look older by thinning the layer of youthful fat beneath her skin. Psychology sweetened her expression, but she said that she couldn't feel happy all the time.

I taught Cynthia Her Luring Brow mov-asana. She was quickly aware of the petulant, irritable, harassed, antisocial look which her tense brows gave her. When she visualized, with sheer willpower, her eyes shifting farther apart from each other, she felt her eye muscles relax, and her brows followed suit. After a little practive (only four days) Cynthia's brows relaxed when she *merely thought* that her eyes were wider apart than they actually were. She felt her scalp, face, neck and upper body relax at the same time, and even her tension headaches vanished.

Cynthia glanced into the mirror and was amazed that she looked no more than 38. Her old friends and acquaintances remarked that she "looked younger every day." Cynthia made new plans for her life. She had never counted on looking so young again!

How to Rid Yourself of Pimples and Other Skin Blemishes

Never have I seen worse cases of acne than in the tropics. Young people in many small retirement towns and their outlying ranches in southern California run the tropical cases a close second. Teenage caucasians who settle in the tropics with their parents frequently break out shockingly with acne. My medical relatives treated numbers of acne patients in the warm climes with startling success. Their treatment, based on Yoga, was simple.

I myself suffered twice from severe acne while in the Canal Zone high school. I treated it by sunbathing for one hour every day and swimming in the Pacific for another hour. Within a week the giant pustules had dried up and turned to scaly tissue which dropped off. (Never peel off that scaly tissue!) I suffered no scars.

This procedure is impractical if you live in a cold climate, particularly inland where the ocean is inaccessible and the sun rays are not intense enough to "cauterize" the pimples. In that event, sponge your face (or the pimples' area) with strong salt water, several times daily. And don't dry it. Let the salt cake over each pustule and draw it to a head.

In the summer, when the sun is hot, lie down on your back and bare your acne to the sun for about one hour. Cover your eyes with a narrow, 2-inch piece of doubled cloth or towel or a plastic eyeballs cover sold in drugstores. Oil the rest of your body for protection.

If your back is pimply, fill three-quarters of your bathtub with tepid water and mix with salt until it tastes like sea-water. Soak your body in it for ten minutes at a time, once a day, for several days.

Another Yoga secret to get rid of acne is: slice a clove of garlic in half and rub the moist pulp on each pimple for about a half minute. Do so before going to bed, so you can rinse off the sulphur odor of the garlic in the morning. You could even tape a tiny piece of sliced off garlic upon the center of the pimple. Either one will bring the pimple to a head, sometimes as early as the very next morning.

Effect of Water on Human Hair

There is little doubt that using water too regularly on your hair dries your scalp and may cause dandruff. If your hair is rather fine in texture and curly, water turns it brittle and unmanageable. If it is coarse and straight, it might lose style.

Brushing—or even combing—your hair daily may cause hair loss, Dr. Norman Orentreich of New York, announced during a recent American Medical Association conference in Chicago, I fully agree. The Yogis believed this for centuries and were called "unkempt" for practicing it. I myself have preached it for two decades. Brushing, no matter how gently done, inflicts trauma upon your hair. Combing your hair regularly is worse. Like the brush, it scrapes your scalp and causes it to thicken in self-defense and strangle the hair follicles. If your hair is curly or wavy, too much combing and brushing breaks it off.

Too frequent washing, other authorities said at the conference, could break hairs, but not produce baldness. In dry areas, though, as in the Southwest and southern California, it may cause dandruff. I found that rubbing the hair dry after wetting it or after swimming stimulates new hair growth. But *don't* comb your hair then. Comb it when it is easiest to comb, such as after a shampoo. When it is "dirty" and you comb it, the comb "tears out" lots of hair. Although the "tearing out" may not cause baldness, it makes your hair look "thin." Keeping your hair "glued" to your scalp in the same position all day weakens its roots and contributes to baldness. Always comb your hair gently, slowly, patiently. Traumatize it, and your scalp, the least possible. Pulling your hair with your fingers, though, but not too hard, strengthens its roots.

An Eastern Method of Encouraging the Growth of Hair

Your hair, like your fingernails and toenails, is not living tissue. But like them, it grows when cut. This is the secret which certain little-known Yogis have used to grow hair back on their balding heads. My own head was alarmingly baldish for ten years before I applied this secret myself and grew back about 85 percent of my hair. This is how to apply this Yogi secret scientifically:

1. Lather with shaving cream the balding area of your scalp.

2. With a safety razor, shave the balding area. (If you aren't self-conscious, shave off all your hair).

3. Shave it again every four days, or as soon as the roots in the balding spot are as stubby as a two or three day old beard.

4. *Do not* shave your head with a barber clip. The edge does not reach the dying roots deeply enough to irritate and stimulate their regrowth.

5. Repeat this procedure for about two to six weeks, if convenient. Repeat it during the same period in the following year, if you wish.

6. All your hair might not grow back, but as much as 90 to 95 percent of it might. Mine practically did! So did that of my dentist uncle, of my first cousin, and of many people to whom I taught the secret.

7. You don't have to massage your scalp unless you want to. Don't even comb or brush the shaved hair stubs. I agree with the Yogis that brushing injures the hair. The sharp ends of the bristles tear your scalp, sandpaper the hair off, and encourage scar tissue to grow over your injured hair follicles and entomb them.

8. Apply no lotion or salve to your shaved scalp. Let the irritated hair follicles remain fully exposed to air and light.

9. Your falling hair will grow back coarser and stronger and—to your astonishment—strikingly thicker! Your friends will stop feeling sorry for you.

10. When outdoors thereafter, wear a hat or a cap to shield your scalp from the sun during the hot hours of the day. The Yogis blame the intense rays of the sun as a leading cause of baldness (and I agree with them). Too much hair grooming is equally to blame. Comb your hair the least possible when you comb it. If it is practical, comb it only once or twice a week. The comb tears out too many roots otherwise. But most people have to comb it every day, of course, for appearance.

A Yoga Protection for Your Teeth

Too many people, including myself, wielded the toothbrush too vigorously for years. So they wore off unnecessarily too much enamel from their teeth, particularly from the bases of their molars and canine teeth where the leverage of the toothbrush handle is most powerful. Dentists used to blame such enamel "erosion" on strong saliva. They know better now. For 40 years my dentist uncle and I blamed it on hard toothbrushes wielded too strongly. I still uphold this assertion, and time will prove me to be right, as it has in so many of my discoveries and conclusions in the psychic and the health field. So, like the Yogis, use no hard toothbrushes. My dentist uncle, though, never had his cleaned though they were very white and clean.

How to Escape Ever-Threatening Gum Diseases

In my book, *Somo-Psychic Power: Using Its Miracle Forces for a Fabulous New Life*, I revealed how the tribal doctor of the Cimarrones, Mormo, saved his gums and his teeth. At 90 they were as young as a youth's. At a recent convention of the American Dental Association held at San Francisco, it was found that 95 percent of the dentists had gum diseases in one form or another, and some had loose teeth. Only 5 percent of them had healthy mouths. Thirty-five percent of them suffered from inflammation of the gums, and 60 percent from diseases of the teeth supporting structures. About 70 percent of American adults, too, suffer from gum diseases.

Two months later, a group of American doctors with Indians in the Panama Canal Zone declared that chewing sugar-cane was fine for the health. The doctors discovered, furthermore, that the cane fibers "clean out food from between the teeth." One of the doctors had even tried it himself.

My prominent dentist uncle in Panama learned this secret from these Indians about 80 years before. (The Yogis have a similar secret.) My uncle used it even after studying dentistry in the United States. In contrast to the dentists at the American Dental Association, in his 80's he still had marvelously healthy gums (and lost only a tooth). He and I concluded, after prolonged microscopic examination in Panama, that the sharp edges of the cut bristles of toothbrushes scraped the soft tissues of the gums even worse than they scraped the hard tissue of the tooth's enamel. Your gums swell gradually over the years from the trauma and bleed until they develop gingivitis. In time, your teeth may loosen. Toothbrushes, we concluded, should be manufactured with natural bristles, or with bristles tapering to soft points.

My uncle would not wait until that was done, if it ever would. So he scrubbed his teeth twice a day with a small cotton ball. He found the cotton to be as smooth and non-abrasive to his gums and enamel as sugar-cane pulp. His teeth and gums, as stated before, remained youthful throughout his long life.

How to Acquire Glamorous Toothshine

The Yogis, as a group, sad to confess, are not particularly proud enough about their teeth. But the Cimarrones (of Darien, Panama) were proud of theirs. They polished them with the fiber of the chewed sugar cane and made them so slick that they shone like blinding lights when they laughed in the sunlight.

You can do likewise with cotton balls as my dentist uncle did. Moisten the small ball of cotton first. Spread ¼-inch of toothpaste on it, and press it hard enough against your teeth to take on their curves. Rub the cotton *away* from your gums, and in that direction only. Use a total of ¼-inch of toothpaste for the whole of *each* of the four non-biting surfaces of all your teeth. These four surfaces are the outer and inner surfaces of your upper teeth and those of your lower teeth. You need less toothpaste for the chewing surfaces of your teeth, or for your tongue, which should be swabbed with the cotton at the end.

Rinse off with a waterpick. Then rub your tongue over your teeth to "feel" whether they are sufficiently clean. Any area that feels rough needs more cleaning. But don't rub it repeatedly and erode the surface of the enamel with hand trauma. Just clean it a little more next time you wash your mouth. Throw away the cotton ball after using it once.

Neither the Cimarrones nor the Yogis use dental floss. The fibers of the mango, when chewed, slip easily between their teeth. But my uncle and I found that dental floss or anything at all that slices between the teeth, lacerated the gums and caused gum trouble. The waterpick, we found, with not too strong a stream, did a fine job and saved the gums from the fine cutting of cleaning fibers.

Important: Avoid sticky foods, like chocolate, which bury into the grooves of your teeth and cause decay. To keep your teeth all your life, eat foods that can be brushed easily off your teeth. It may also be advisable to have your teeth cleaned with ultra-sound about once a year, unless your dentist advises differently.

How to Save Your Gums from the Effects of Destructive Emotions

Some experts believe that extreme or prolonged emotion brought on by extreme or simple social stress constricts the blood vessels of your gums and thereby break down your gums. This may very well be true, too. The gentle massage which the cotton gives your gums without scraping them should greatly overcome this possible cause.

Chewing gum, it has been found in Sweden, does not remove plaque, nor stop the accumulation of plaque on your teeth.

The American Dental Association advises you to eat less sweets between meals, to brush your teeth back-and-forth instead of up and down, to use a brush with soft bristles, and to use a fluoride toothpaste. Such counselling is of the utmost value. But it is difficult to find a very soft, natural bristled toothbrush. When it is too soft, besides, the bristles bend and push under your gums and irritate them and pack bacteria beneath them. I still insist that cotton is better, and to brush your teeth with it only in *one* direction: that is, *away* from your gums *to* the biting surfaces of your teeth. Your gums are traumatized the least by the "brushing" then, and bacteria is not packed into their edges. And, of course, eat nothing between meals, not even sweets or sweet drinks.

How to Protect Your Vision from Your Ruinous Environment (ten scientific Yoga secrets)

Even if you never abuse your eyes, your unsuspectedly ruinous environment can ruin your eyesight. From arising to bedtime your eyes are being half-blinded by the traumas of light reflections of all sorts. Even highly-polished furnishings in your home or office, as well as reflections from mirrors, magnify the irritant power of the light striking them and drive it into your eyes with an intensity that traumatizes your retina and your optic nerves.

1. *On the street* your eyes are assailed by reflections from the sun from the windows of high-rise buildings when the sun rays strike the window glass at certain angles. . .
By reflections:

off the plated surfaces on the front of your car and of other vehicles on the sunny days. . .

from the street itself about 20 to 30 feet ahead of you when the sun is strong. . .

from the guiding mirror, if you are the one driving. . . and even from the inside of your car when the sun rays flash into it from a low angle.

2. *In your office* your eyes are assailed by the overhead light as it reflects off the smooth glass, or the flat top, of your polished desk. . .

from the frosted glass door if there is a strong overhead light. . .

from cars passing by on the street when you sit in a restaurant for lunch, either facing or sitting sideways to the street, or when you stroll through the street.

3. *On your way home from work*, particularly in the cooler months with their shorter days, most cars put on their lights early. These scour your eyes all the way home. These lights are even more merciless to your eyes when you drive at night.

4. *After dinner* you probably read with a low-set lamp before you or at eye level somewhere in the room. It batters still more your all-day suffering eyes.

If you work or read under a fluorescent lamp, the rays are more evenly distributed; but their all-around glare stuns your sight.

If you watch TV regularly, the rays from the screen irritate your eyes still further, especially if it is a black-and-white set. But if it is a color set, the extra and different radiation has been known to cause cancer. Protect your eyes from TV glare by keeping the illumination dial turned low, or by simply wearing lightly tinted sunglasses when you watch it.

5. *When you go boating or fishing* the reflection of the sun off the water can blind you eventually. Columbus and several of his sailors lost their sight from them. I know several persons of leisure who turned blind merely from taking long daily health walks for years without protecting their eyes with sunglasses or wide brimmed hats. Others have developed cataracts. If there is a parking place within seeing distance from where you boat or fish, as there is in most recreation areas, the reflections of the sun off the numerous windshields as the sun moves across the sky can blind you temporarily—and even permanently—in the course of time.

Even the silverware on your table, if it is under a harsh or low-standing light, can traumatize your sight to a degree. Wearing sunglasses in the daytime, and driver's glasses at night, are about the only protection you have against the traumas described in the preceeding paragraph. When walking, standing, or sitting outdoors and the wind is light, you can add or substitute the sunglasses with a wide-brimmed hat. But you can't drive a vehicle safely wearing such a hat, for it might interfere with your view. Drive less at night, if you can help it. The trauma of sunshine to your eyes in the daytime is no less severe than that of the bright night lights. Strong street lights help the driver and the pedestrian, but they also destroy your eyes.

6. *Reading or writing* on a flat desk distorts the shape of your lens in your effort to see more clearly. To save your eyes, hold or set up the reading material always *closely parallel to your face*, such as in the position in which you hold the paper when you read it on the bus, train, or plane. Rest the reading matter against a support and leave your arms free to write or turn the pages, instead of letting

them cramp holding up the material. Cramped, tired arms, besides, reduce your reading efficiency. Waste the least amount of energy, in other words, when you sit back and read. Let the light itself reflect upon the pages from high enough behind you, over your right shoulder. When the source of the light is too close to you, even if behind you, it reflects too much glare off the pages or object in your hands. It also heats your scalp excessively, damaging your hair follicles.

7. *Write* on a desk surface that rises away from you at an angle of about 30 degrees from the ground. When you bend over normally to write, the desk surface will then be almost parallel to your sight. Typing is far less strenuous than writing because the letters you type on the page are practically parallel to your eyes. Being far more legible, too, they strain your eyes less when you read them. Writing in long- or shorthand traumatizes your eyes badly because the lens of your eyes focus upon the thin, moving lines of the letters as you scribble them. While, when you type, the keys print whole, formed letters instead of thin, moving lines. They, thus, alter the shape of your lens less to read them. Following the needle while sewing, as with forming thin lines, is also brutal to your eyes.

8. *Stop all reading or writing* for about seven to eight minutes straight every hour and get up and walk around to rest your eyes. Even do something physical which needs to be done, or as much of it as you can during that interval. Your buttocks regain circulation then, too, which helps to prevent constipation—and prostate trouble, if you are a man. Indeed, it is wise to massage your hips with your hands for a minute or two, or longer, as you walk about at this time, to encourage more blood to flow into your pelvic-blocked area. If you are a man, this will help you still more to avoid prostate trouble, or to improve it if you already have it.

9. *Rest your eyes* after reading for three hours by lying down on your back if you have the opportunity. Cover your eyes with a dark lightweight material even if you are in a dark room to relieve the retinas from adjusting to the least glare.

10. I myself was in first grade at the age of four. I have read, studied, researched, and written all my life since then. I have written tens of millions of words—and I am still writing and note-taking. Although at 30 I was prescribed glasses, I have hardly worn them, and still wear them very little. So, with the help of the Yogi secrets, I protect my eyes against the ruinous environment.

Five Yoga Secrets to Guard Against and Improve Cataracts

The Yogis are constantly threatened with cataracts. Cataracts are most prevalent in hot, sunny climates. They result from years of exposing the lens to the daily traumas of intense heat and light, such as that of the Indian deserts. Blue-eyed people develop cataracts even in cold climates if they don't wear sunglasses and take other precautions.

The Yogi, for that reason, is cataract conscious. Out there in the wilderness, blindness or very poor sight is equivalent to death, which it soon brings. Here are the Yogi secrets, made scientific, to guard against, and improve, cataract:

1. The Yogi sits with his back to the sun. When he faces the sun he limits it to a short period in the very early morning and rotates his head to "sun" every seeing region of his retina and re-enforce it against the expected daily traumas of daylight. But this practice is not recommended for most people. During World War II a number of servicemen in a Texas camp for months stared at the sun every morning to "strengthen" their eyes. Many went blind or suffered permanent losses of parts of their sights. Never, for that reason, sit with a "reflector" beaming sunlight back into your face either, as some people ignorantly do at many beaches.

2. Don't stare across a body of water which reflects the sun. Don't even stand at the edge of water which reflects the sun back up into your eyes. It is commonly known, as stated before, that Columbus and many of his sailors eventually went blind from the daily reflections of the sun from the surface of the ocean, from which their comparatively small, low-deck vessels protected them little.

3. Don't spend too much time a day near ovens or other extremely hot objects. The lens of your eyes are composed of albumen (a protein), like the white of an egg. Excessive heat over the years can coagulate it, just as heat does to the white of an egg. That is precisely what a cataract is. And you can't see through a coagulated lens.

4. When you walk in the sun, make sure that it shines upon you from in back. If it shines into your eyes from the front, or from the top or side of you into your eyes regularly for hours a day, many months during the year, you risk developing cataract, particularly of the lens most directly "struck" by the sun. Wearing a hat helps, but the brim has to be broad enough to shield the whole of your eyes from the sun. Americans in the tropics who wear hats have still developed cataracts in the lower halves of their lens where the hat-brims did not throw shadows. Too, people who stroll in the mid-afternoon with the sun shining regularly more on one side of them have developed cataracts of the lens of that side, and none, or less, of the lens of their other side.

5. The same applies to reflections from windshields, windows of high-rises near or far, "plated" parts of cars, from the surfaces of highways if you travel long distances in hot, dry weather, from night lights on the road or from cars, from excessive heat or lights in your own residence.

Wearing a hat with a wide brim when you go outdoors for an hour or more is an effective way as explained to escape cataract induced by the sun. In windy regions, though, you might have to fasten the hat down, or it will blow off easily.

Note: Wearing a hat that tends to blow from your head causes your frontalis muscles (the muscles of your brows) to contract as your forehead instinctively tries to "hang on" to the hat. That reflex will wrinkle your forehead prematurely. So, it is wiser to fasten your hat down in a windy place with an attachment going under your chin. Or keep it on with the hood of an outdoor garment if the weather is cool.

A final word. If you are already afflicted with a degree of cataract, these precautions can help your lens regain a varying degree of normalcy. Although eggwhite never returns to a liquid once it jells, I know several persons who regained different degrees of normal vision by taking the precautions of the Yoga secrets. They also had full faith that the precautions would work. Medical experimenters themselves admit now that people with faith in their treatments recover more easily and completely than those without it.

How Anton D. Saw Much Better Than He Had for Years

Anton D. was growing desperate because his eyes seemed to see less clearly, although his vision still tested normal. But he had a few cataract spots and feared that they would grow and block out his sight.

Anton applied the Yoga secrets which I had made scientific. He "hated" to wear a hat, he told me, but persisted. He kept away from exposures to intense heat and discontinued his annual vacations to hot climate paradises. He grew super-aware of excessive light reflections and turned his back to them whenever he could, or closed his eyes, or departed from the area.

In a few months he noticed a decided change in his vision. In two years he insisted that he saw more clearly than he had since he was a young man. His eyes, further, had lost their redness and strained look. The whites were clear and shiny, and the lines under his eyes were gone.

Yoga Ways to Save Your Hearing Year After Year

Guard your hearing every day, or your auditory nerve will lose its acuity and leave you deaf or partly deaf in your advancing years. Noise from all around you bombards your ears at every breath. Many noises emanate from airplanes, traffic, construction, garbage recycling, high winds, subways, crowds, stereos, typewriters, modern music. You have little cooperative protection against them because noisy products sell better than quiet ones. The buying public, market psychologists found, believe that the noisy products are more powerful and efficient than the quiet ones. Manufacturers who made quiet airplanes, can openers, vacuum cleaners, electric typewriters, jack-hammers and other machines lost money.

If you can do nothing else when trapped in the noise, lightly press the tips of your index fingers in your ears. If possible, stay far from the noise area. If you are indoors, shut your windows tight if you can. Plug your ears with Swedish cotton and, to protect your ears from rupturing, open your mouth to neutralize the sound waves. Target practice, of course, is noisy—as well as poisonous, for it releases gunpowder in the air. So is motor-boating. To plug your ears for hours at a time is neither comfortable nor healthy. It blocks fresh air from entering your auditory canal. But it is better to resort to it than to be prematurely deafened, or to be deafened at all. Ignore people who laugh at you for protecting your ears. They laughed at me most of my life for exercising, and for making psychic discoveries which the scientific world is at long last, from one to 30 years later, proving to be true. Highway construction workers are driven deaf by repeated noise from heavy machinery. They don't protect their ears because their co-workers call that "sissified." But, better to be called a sissy than to turn deaf. Protect your ears, likewise, from machines which you yourself use, either at home or at your work. Also avoid hobbies which create too much noise and imperil your hearing.

5

How Yoga Can Overcome
the Symptoms of Chronic Ailments

Bringing Your Physiological Rhythms Under Control

Your physiological (circadian) rhythms would be all but *un*detectable if your adrenal glands were removed. This proves that your sympathetic nervous system, by affecting the dynamism of your adrenal glands, controls your circadian rhythms, or your daily hormonal secretion rhythms. When your circadian rhythm is out of control, you are a negative person when you should be positive, and a positive person when you should be negative. You are then victimized by your emotions and are converted into a chaotic, vastly inferior person who fails at practically everything you attempt.

For thousand of years, though, the Yogis have changed their own brain waves, heart rates, blood pressures, and other "automatic" functions. Researchers in numerous medical centers all across the United States finally admit it and are trying to teach it to ordinary people in all walks of life, using electrical "alpha-wave" machines. They even agree that it can be taught to people "frequently without machinery or electrical devices," admits a university clinical psychologist, Dr. Daniel Logan, University of Texas Southwestern Medical School (in 1973.)[1]

The Yogis have always learned how, and taught it to their adepts, without machinery or electrical devices. Their secret to stabilize your circadian rhythms is the Di-urnal Swing-Ho mov-asana. Use it to keep yourself under self-control and remain a fully integrated, self-ruling person. Here is how to do it. (Follow Figure 17.)

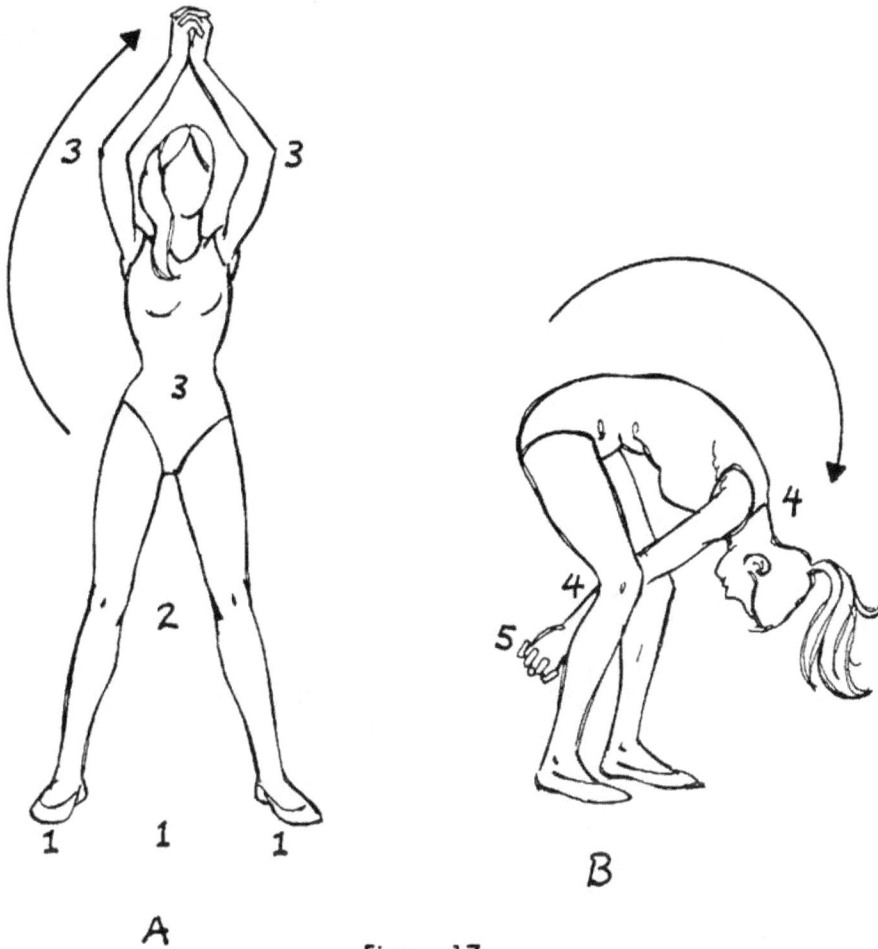

Figure 17
The Di-urnal Swing-Ho

The Marvel of the Diurnal Swing-Ho

The position to assume (Figure 17A)

1. Stand with your heels from 15 to 18 inches apart, depending on your height. Let your toes point normally slightly outwards.

2. Have knees nearly straight.

3. Inhale. Bend your arms. Raise them above your head and fold your hands into each other.

How to do this Yoga mov-asana (Figure 17B)

4. Exhale. Bend your knees, and bend forward, and

5. Swing your joined arms down between your knees, as far back as you can.

6. Reassume the position in Number 1, and repeat.

Frequency: 10 times. 1 set (group of repetitions) once a day. But, if you wish, do 2 or 3 sets of 10 repetitions each. Rest 10 seconds between sets.

How to Swing-Ho this Yoga mov-asana

1. Do the movement vigorously, as if chopping wood in a country paradise.

2. As you progress down the repetitions from 1 to 10, your back will stretch, and your arms will consequently swing farther and farther back between your legs.

What the Diurnal Swing-Ho does for you:

1. Brings your circadian rhythms more under control. Throws the laggard ones out of their lethargy, and activates the "wayward" ones to synchronize with them. Bending your lower back, too, where your adrenal glands are located, stimulates the dynamism of these glands into controlling your daily hormonal secretion rhythms. You then fall into stride with your best natural physiological cycle.

2. With the chopping wood action you "let off steam." You can then control your emotions much easier during your active hours.

3. Wears off excess flesh from your lower back, and some from your sides.

4. Fills your brain with fresh new blood.

How Leo Z. "Let off Steam" and Enjoyed His Work

Leo Z. felt listless and disinterested in everything, particularly his work. He dreaded going to it and resented every moment he spent at it. He didn't feel like himself in anything he did, in fact, as if his mind and body were beating off-key. He was impelled to throw everything overboard and flee somewhere and live "like a bum." He couldn't get himself together. Nobody he went to could help him, he said.

I taught Leo The Diurnal Swing-Ho. In his very first "workout" he felt a "venomous steam" shoot out of him. Immediately thereafter, his mind and body, "for once," seemed to beat *on* key. Something "out-of-line" in him had suddenly adjusted to the rest of him and *harmonized his whole person*. As an additional blessing, he felt his lower back stretch decisively. It was losing its ugly fat! Leo called the mov-asana "the next thing to magic. . . and so easy and pleasant to do!"

The Causes of Many Different Headaches

Here are 13 different kinds of headaches and their causes. Find out which is yours.

1. Caffeine is a strong stimulant and causes your stomach to secrete gastric juice of high acidity. So is beer, alcohol, liver extract, meat, vegetable extracts.

2. All these causes, in time, enlarge your stomach glands and turn your stomach chronically acid. You are saddled, as a result, with a constant headache, or with off-and-on headaches, depending upon the concentration of the acid created. Such a headache feels to you as if someone is hammering or pressing down near the top of your head with an iron pole.

3. Alcohol dilates the blood vessels of the covering of your brain, triggering a headache over the whole area of your brain: the well-known "hang-over."

4. Caffeine in larger doses retards the circulation of blood to your brain. The amount of oxygen carried to your brain is thereby reduced, causing pain in the same manner as less oxygen in your muscles when you exercise causes the pain of cramps. The pain is the silent call of your muscles for more oxygen.

5. Nicotine dilates your blood vessels. So your heart speeds up to bring your resulting lower blood pressure back to normal. Too much blood is then rushed to your brain, stretching the nerve endings of the nerves of pain in it and causing a headache.

6. Eating too many meals, eating too frequently, or too much, also turn your stomach "acid."[2] As a result, too much blood is drawn from your head and muscles to your stomach to digest your food, leaving too little blood for your head, causing headaches.

7. Exercising too soon after eating causes a partial indigestion that results in headaches.[3]

8. Drinking too little water does not reduce sufficiently the acid in your stomach and can result in headaches.[4]

9. Eating chocolate (the darker variety, especially) can afflict you with headache because it is concentrated food, not easy to digest, and overstimulates your stomach glands.[5]

10. Too much fresh air (such as from deep breathing too frequently or too consecutively and thus driving off too much "impure" air from your lungs) can give you headaches because your brain temporarily stops calling for more oxygen. Your brain needs some impure air (some carbon dioxide instead of oxygen) in it to incite it to call for oxygen.

11. Excessive hunger between meals indicates too much acid in your stomach, which can result in a headache. Neutralize the acidity by drinking *plain water* between meals.[6] *Don't drink fruit juices between meals!*[7] Their delightful taste and molecular-bulk content only stimulate your stomach glands to secrete *still more* acid, thus increasing your stomach acidity.

12. Too much staring at TV strains your retina (the seeing surface within your eyes) and causes headaches.[8] A poor reading lamp causes too much blood to be drawn to your retina to form photographic images, thus causing headache.

13. Eating too much acid-forming concentrated foods, like cheese, nuts, and candies, can bring on headaches. They cause your stomach to secrete too much gastric juice to moisten and digest them.

How to Avoid Avoidable Headaches (Eight Secrets)

Here are the Yoga secrets with which to avoid different kinds of headaches.

1. Eat three regular meals a day, *no more*.

2. Drink only water between meals. It will reduce the acid in your stomach by neutralizing a part of it. It also fills your stomach and reduces your between-meals appetite.

3. When your stomach is empty, do Your Super-Mind Awakener (page 191), Your Diurnal Swing-Ho (page 85), or assume their lowered postures for a few seconds at a time. They will drive more oxygen-carrying blood to your brain and wash out the stagnating blood. When you stand up straight again, the blood to your brain will be normal.

4. Do a vigorous Yoga mov-asana like Your Neck-Shoulder Line Perfecter (page 62), to stimulate your sympathetic nervous system and accelerate the blood circulation to your brain. The stagnating blood in your brain will be forced out and carried to your lungs to be oxygenated. Non-Yoga exercises which are also highly recommended to stop headaches are jogging, sprinting, fast swimming.

5. Drink four glasses of water one after another. Repeat it an hour later. The hyperacidity in your stomach will be reduced speedily.

6. Eat, for a whole week, a thick slice of watermelon at breakfast.

7. Never go to bed on a full stomach. Wait about three hours after a heavy meal, and two hours after a light one. Ignore the derision of the stubborn, reckless, or ignorant.

8. If all these means fail, see your physician or healer, if you didn't before. Your atlas, the first vertebra in your neck, might need adjusting.

Loosening Your Muscles to Relax Your Nerves

Don't ignore pain as a matter of principle. When it is not muscular, it may be the warning signal of some serious condition in your body. But when a diagnosis indicates that your pain is simply a bothersome or nagging one which you are advised to tolerate (such as, from arthritis, synovitis, bursitis, strained joints, sciatica, and other conditions which don't heal quickly), no Yogi would advise you to resort to tranquilizers, braces, anesthetic injections, or to any other non-natural means—unless you are being treated by a professional healer. Such pain relievers weaken your muscles or joints, or flood your system with drugs that mask the pain but undermine your health and leave you at the mercy of other ailments or diseases. It is wiser to control your pain without them.

Heat and ice packs, both, when applied to your painful areas, reduce the pain, although for the opposite reasons. Heat increases the flow of blood through your painful part and removes the waste accumulating in it, the acidity of which is the cause of the pain. Ice packs, on the other hand, chill the nerve endings in the painful part, thus preventing them from conveying the pain messages to your brain.

But it is impractical to apply hot or cold applications to your painful area when you are outside your home or at work. You *can* reduce the intensity of the pain you feel, however, by simply relaxing. When you are calm, your brain evaluates the pain messages it receives from your painful part, with much less intensity. When you are tense or jittery, in contrast, your brain *exaggerates* the pain messages it receives from your painful part. Much of the agony from which you suffer when nervous and over-wrought, for example, vanishes when you relax. When your mind is deeply engrossed in other matters, in fact, it even ignores altogether the pain messages it receives from any part of you. A boxer fighting with a broken jaw or knuckle, who hardly feels pain until after the contest, is a striking instance.

That is the secret of why the Yogi feels no pain, even when strapped down upon a bed of sharp nails, or with a pin stuck through his cheek or arm. You yourself can acquire that power. That is the Yogi's secret, made scientific. Here is the mov-asana for you to acquire a similar power to serve you daily in emergencies.

1. Clench your fists tightly.

2. Hold them clenched for five seconds, or until your forearm muscles start to pain you. Then

3. Relax your fists completely by extending your fingers fully. Your forearm muscles will stop paining you fast.

4. Clench your fists tightly again. Imagine this time that a *painful part* of your body has been *transferred* to your *forearms*. Feel your forearms hurt as much as the painful part, in other words, but "feel" the painful part itself hurt *no more*.

5, Relax your fists completely again by extending your fingers all the way. This time, though, feel all the transferred pain in your forearms leave them through your hands and fingers INTO THE AIR.

That is how the Yogi controls *any pain* in his body with hardly a move. He just loosens his muscles to relax his nerves. Master this easy pain-transferring Yogi secret and free yourself from pain *anytime, anywhere*, by merely clenching and unclenching your fists.

Guarding from, or Relieving, the Discomfort of Varicose Veins

The constant downpull of gravity when you are standing, in action or weight-bearing, particularly when your leg muscles are weary, overburdens the veins of your legs. Those on the outer surface suffer the most and can turn varicose (that is, abnormally and irregularly swollen or dilated). The harder the ground, the worse the effect, as described in my book *Yoga For Men Only.*[9] The Yogis have long known this and take many precautions to avoid or relieve varicose veins.

While he was Chancellor of Chicago University, Robert Hutchins was asked if he exercised. He replied cryptically, "I sit when I don't have to stand, and I lie down when I don't have to sit." As far as guarding from, or relieving, the discomforts of varicose veins is concerned, the principle could not be stated better. But since you can't always avoid standing, nor can you always lie down when you don't have to sit, there are other precautions to follow. Here they are:

When standing, try not to stand on one leg too long. Don't stand with both legs stiff, for that slows down the circulation to both legs. But don't throw your weight on one leg, either, and strain its blood vessels. Stand on both legs at the same time, but have both knees bent slightly, though not noticeably. The slight bend prevents the blood from flowing perpendicularly down your legs and permits your anti-gravity muscles to relax just enough to slacken their pressure tension against the arteries and veins of your legs. Try to get off your feet at every opportunity, as Robert Hutchins declared he did, and sit, even for a short spell. If that is impossible, stroll around a little to save your legs from being kept in one straining position too long.

Don't walk, run, jog, climb, or engage in any activity on your legs repeatedly for so long at a time that it exhausts them and fills them with excessive blood that over-dilates their arteries and veins. I don't recommend wearing support hose, unless prescribed by your doctor or healer. It does squeeze your leg veins and helps prevent the upflowing blood in them from dropping back in them and straining their closed valves. Simultaneously, though, it also squeezes your arteries and capillaries and forces the downflowing blood in them *back up* into your heart and strains it! It is wiser to follow the Yogi secrets described in this section (unless you are following your healer's orders) and avoid wearing support hose.

How the Yogi Lays His Hands on Varicosing Veins

If spidery veins of strain are showing or start showing on your legs, rub your fingers, when you lie down, gently over them a few times in direction towards your heart. It will encourage the stagnated blood to move on instead of remaining in the veins and stretching them further and weakening their valves still more. I have known many persons, including myself, who have made these forming "spiders" practically disappear in a few months. Such gentle rubbing acts the same as support hose, except that you exert the pressure more on the stretching superficial veins and much less upon the deeper lying arteries. Repeat this several times during your active day to help your overstretched blood vessels.

Holding cold packs against these varicosing parts or immersing your legs in very cold water also helps to reduce these veins. (Water below 50 degrees F., though, it has been found, may cause blood clots.[10]) Never, just the same, exercise violently on your feet in hot weather or in a hot atmosphere if your veins are turning varicose.

How to Free Yourself from Foot Miseries Forever

Your feet are strained by excessive daily standing and improper use, such as, from driving your car, wearing stylish but injuriously designed shoes, walking on hard floors or pavements, lack of enough exercise, habitually standing and using elevators and moving stairs instead of climbing steps, repetitious trauma in such sports as golf, tennis, handball, billiards, bowling, skiing, skating, dancing, jogging, sprinting, or walking, or from insufficient use, as in swimming or bicycling. Your feet are weakened, strained, or partially crippled in time. (A prominent author of animal books was handicapped for 20 years before he died of arthritis of the feet resulting from playing tennis for years on hard courts for long periods at a time). With tender feet, much of your daily pleasure and efficiency vanishes. The symptoms of aging show on your face and in your discontented demeanor.

Strengthen your feet easily and cheaply with the Yoga Calf-Raise mov-asana. (Follow Figure 18.)

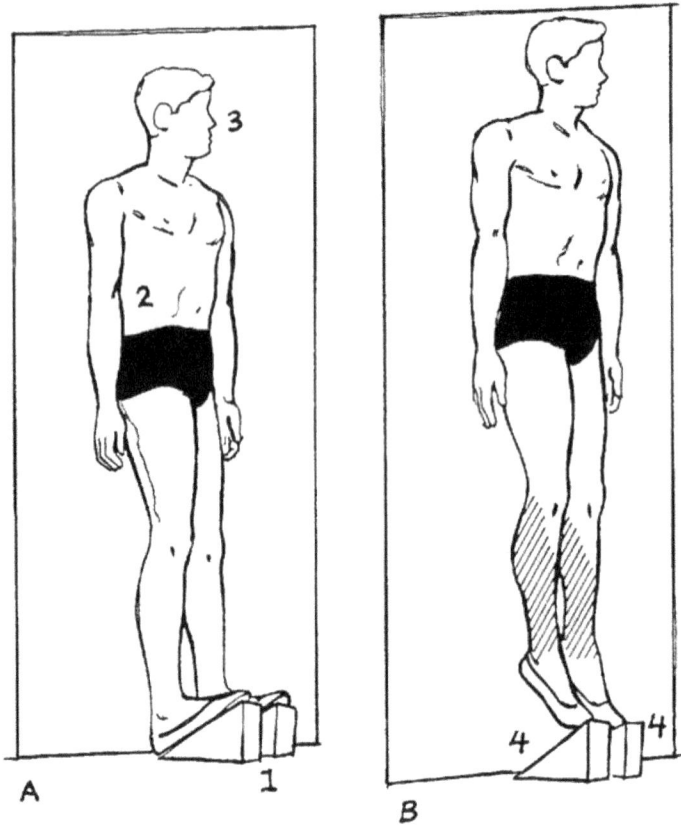

Figure 18
The Yoga Calf-Raise

The position to assume (Figure 18A)

1. Set two triangular blocks close to a partition, or corner of a doorway, parallel to each other, hip-width apart. Point the high ends away from the wall.

2. Stand with your back against the wall, with your feet flat on the blocks. Your toes will lie several inches higher than your heels.

3. Look directly ahead of you to keep your back straight.

How to do this Yoga mov-asana (Figure 18B)

4. Raise your body up and down at a medium pace (about two raises per second). Push up from the balls of your feet.

5. Repeat ten times.

6. Step off the blocks. Walk around for about ten seconds to relax your calves. Then repeat.

Frequency: 10 repetitions. 3 sets (groups of repetitions). Eventually, raise the repetitions to 20 or 30.

What The Yoga Calf-Raise mov-asana does for you.

1. Strengthens your ankles and insteps.

2. Develops or fills out the inner muscles of your calves (your soleus muscles) and removes the long-ankled look, if you have one.

3. Your feet feel springy and alive. Soon, long standing will hardly bother them, although you should avoid subjecting them to such trauma.

4. Jogging or using your legs strenuously in any occupation or sport will fatigue you much less.

5. You will feel considerably younger and happier—or like your "old self" again.

6. *Don't* do this mov-asana with weights in your hands. If you are overweight, do less repetitions. If you are underweight, do more. But don't exceed 12 repetitions a set.

How a Yogi Uses Psychic Electrosleep to Revitalize His Powers

Many Yogis have long been noted for their fantastic trances in which they hibernate sometimes up to 40 days, buried underground, or dash for 100 miles over rough terrain without stopping. Russian scientists are now reproducing this type of trance with electrically-induced relaxation, called "electrosleep," to treat insomnia, ulcers, high blood pressure, and anxiety. It relaxes patients by soothing their brains with a tingling electric current. The sessions last about a half-hour and are carried on five days a week, sometimes extending over several months. Nearly all the sessions are combined with a period of psychotherapy.

The Yogis, though, achieved their equivalent "electrosleep" without electrodes applied over their brows and behind their ears or anywhere else on their bodies. There is no certainty, after all, that other individuals or you might not suffer undesirable side effects after an outside current passes through your brain. People have!

But you *can* fall *safely* into a self-induced electrosleep (or psychic electrosleep) and help yourself overcome many ailments, including sleeplessness, ulcers, high blood pressure, and anxiety. Here is the Yoga secret for falling into such a sleep.

1. Sit back comfortably and hum a sound. Keep humming and

2. Let your neck relax forwards and fall gently towards your chest.

3. The pitch of your voice goes down.

4. *That* is *your* self-inducing sleep voice—your Sleep Mantra Sound.

5. *Listen to it well.*

6. Then practice and reproduce it at will.

How to fall asleep at any time

7. Whenever you wish to fall asleep thereafter, imagine yourself surrounded by an electromagnetic field of total slumber.

8. Relax, then, and hum your Sleep Mantra Sound. Its pitch will go down, and your hearing will dull.

9. You will soon fall asleep.

How Helen U. Felt Fully-Refreshed Every Morning

Helen U. seldom felt rested in the mornings because she seldom slept soundly at night. She went to bed on time regularly, but lay awake for hours recalling her troubles. By morning her head felt heavy and bloated.

I taught Helen how to produce Her Sleep Mantra Sound. She seemed to suffer from an undiagnosable muscle-restlessness-induced anxiety. I have detected this mysterious condition in the patients of many doctors and chiropractors, as well as in hundreds of people in both Americas.

Helen found Her Sleep Mantra Sound mov-asana exciting. On the third night that the pitch of her humming voice went down and her hearing dulled, she fell promptly asleep. (Several others to whom I taught the secret fell asleep *the very first time* they tried it.)

Helen slept soundly regularly thereafter and, in a few weeks, felt and looked 15 years younger. Her work efficiency increased remarkably. She became so full of energy that she even enrolled in night school to qualify for a very attractive promotion.

Secret Ritual to Get Rid of Sore Throat

Sore throat due to strep infection is an inflammation of the mucous membrane of your throat which spreads into your windpipe (trachea). The old "shot of whisky" remedy is fallacious because when you drink alcohol it *bypasses* your windpipe and pours down into your stomach instead.

The easiest way to reach your sore throat is through your throat itself.

Take one-half glass of tepid water.

Mix a heaping teaspoonful of salt in it (or make the salt mixture as strong as sea-water).

Stand up and take a *tiny* portion of the salt water in your mouth.

Drop your head back, until your nose points nearly straight up to the ceiling. But *don't strain* your neck.

Gargle the tiny portion of salt water in your throat. Gargle it gently—*so gently* that the water fits into the opening of your windpipe and almost gags you. Let the salt water, in brief, assume the closest contact possible with the inflamed membranes of your throat and windpipe. Let out the smallest flow of air from your windpipe, in order to gargle the salt water as long as you can.

Spit out the salt water, and gargle with more of it.

After six or seven such gargles, bend far down over the sink and *softly* cough out the loosened mucous matter.

If there is enough space where you live and you feel mildly acrobatic, set your hands on the floor, about one foot from your wall, and kick your feet up against the wall. (Stand on your hands, in other words, with your heels resting against the wall.) In that position, softly cough out still more loosened mucous matter. *Much more* of it will be dislodged.

Repeat the gargling five to six times a day for two days. But don't gargle for one hour after a meal. And don't ''handstand'' against the wall before two and one-half to three hours after a meal.

Caution: Try to swallow *none*, or very little, of the salt water, or it will give you gas. Immediately after each gargling session, finish by gargling once with a tiny portion of plain water deep down your throat, and spit it out. You will swallow some of the salt water each time, otherwise.

How to end your sore throat even faster

If you are staying home from work for a day or two, take two cloves of garlic, each about the mass of about one-third of your little finger. Finely slice them and mix the pieces in your breakfast salad. Do likewise with your supper salad. As stated before, garlic contains three enemies of germs: nitrogen, sulphur, and iodine. Penicillium contains only two of them: nitrogen and sulphur. Garlic for that reason, as the Russians have proved, is more effective than penicillium as a germ abater. Its fumes, in addition, are exhaled from your bloodstream into your windpipe when they leave your lungs, and suffocate the bacteria in your throat. Penicillium releases no such fumes. That's why it has no healing smell.

How to end your sore throat faster still

The Yogis have demonstrated, contrary to popular belief, that vigorous exercise is a drastic enemy of sore throat. So, sprint *as fast as you can* each day you suffer from sore throat for a short distance, depending upon your physical condition. Immediately afterwards, walk three times that distance, and sprint again! Such full power exertion will awaken your sympathetic nervous system to a pugnacious degree and raise your body temperature to a germ-slaughtering level. (The "shot of whisky" will also raise your body temperature, but you may have to drink it a number of times, or enough to harm yourself in some other manner.)

At the end of each sprint, stop and bend over. Place your hands on your knees, with your elbows bent halfway to support your body. Then gently dislodge the loosened mucous with your heavy breathing and spit it out. (For community hygienic reasons it is best to spit it out into a paper handkerchief that can be flushed away in the toilet.)

This natural, scientific Yoga mov-asana is so effective that, even if you still eat sweets and starchy foods, it will still knock out your sore throat. It is wiser, of course, to avoid such foods for a week or two, for they probably help to bring on your sore throat in the first place. But don't fast, go on a liquid diet, or weaken yourself resting in bed or taking hot baths for days. Don't even take therapeutic doses of vitamin C on your own and risk developing kidney stones.

After sprinting and walking from five to 15 minutes altogether, rest at home from one-half to one hour. Follow these directions closely for three or four days and you will feel as strong as a bull.

How to Break up a Head Cold and Sinusitis with Yoga

The Yogis break up head colds in much the same manner as they get rid of sore throats (described previously). But instead of gargling with salted water, they draw it in *gently* through their nostrils and gently blow it out again. This is the Yoga mov-asana way, made scientific, to do it:

1. Fill a small, two or three-inch deep, plastic basin with water. Mix the water with salt until it is strong enough—or as strong as sea water. (But no stronger than that).

2. Hold the basin over your washroom sink and bend over, at the waist, and place your nose in the water.

3. Inhale the water gently. If your nose is stopped up, very little water will seep into it at first. But the warm salt water will permeate the blocking mucous

matter and liquify and dislodge it and bring out most of it through your nose, and some of it through your mouth.

4. After doing the aforementioned two or three times, put the basin down and blow your nose *gently*. *Blow* with both nostrils and your mouth open. (This is the *Yogi* way.) "Ease out the dislodged mucous plug," to be exact. Don't force out any of the obstructing mucous with air power, or the mucous could be jammed into your inner ear and threaten you with middle ear infection. Let such resistant mucous wait until the next time you do this mov-asana.

5. Now, prepare some more salt water in a glass and gargle your throat and mouth to rinse out any remaining loose mucous which may have lodged in your throat and spread the infection.

6. Repeat the whole process next morning, up to four mornings. But don't inhale the salt water into your nose more than two times each morning.

7. Carry a paper handkerchief with you all day, because your nose may be ready to be blown one or two hours later, and get rid of more dislodged mucous. *Gently* blow this matter out, again with *both* nostrils and your mouth open.

8. Follow the other directions for fighting off Sore Throat. Your nose will be clear in a few days—and without fasting or drugging yourself.

Yoga Secret for a Reverberating Voice

Your unbalanced daily diet, the daily bad air and environmental pollution, your natural elimination of metabolic waste products, even the debris of the bacteria in your nasal passages, form a blanket of mucous over the floors of your sinuses which contribute, day and night, to various degrees of post-nasal drip. This drip glues itself over your vocal chords and robs your voice of its natural timbre. On the floor of your sinuses, too, it reduces your voice resonance and deprives you of one of the most effective daily instruments for success in life, especially if you deal with the public in person or by telephone. It also lessens your mental acuity, for it makes your brain feel somewhat dull, as if you are not totally "clear" in the head. If you can rid yourself of this daily plague, your voice would boom with surprising power and conviction, even when you speak softly. And your head would feel so light, and your mind would be so youthfully alert, that you would succeed as you never have before socially, romantically, and in business.

The Yoga secret to achieve this "miracle success" instrument is simple. Just irrigate your nasal cavity (and therefore, your frontal sinuses) every morning upon arising with warm salt water, as the Yogis do for a head cold. Inhale the salt water through your nose five times. Sniff or spit it out each time, gently. Some of it will still drip from your nose a half-hour later, but just blow it out gently.

The rest of the day you will be a *totally different person!* It is also a tremendous protection against catching colds or sore throat.

If you prefer, you can do it at night, at bedtime, especially if you have a thin face, for any kind of nasal irrigation leaves the face looking a bit thinner or strained for about three hours afterwards. But don't skip a day! This is a truly magical Yoga secret!

Lifting Pressure off Your Neck Nerves

Your shoulders are held up by muscles that attach to your neck and skull. The downpull of gravity on your shoulders fatigues these muscles and throws them into spasm. As a result, they squeeze the nerves and blood vessels lying close to them and diminish the amount of normal oxygen being brought to your brain to feed it. Your memory, your creativity, your power of concentration, and the even balance between your sympathetic and parasympathetic nervous systems are disturbed by it. Lift the pressure off your neck nerves and return your brain functions

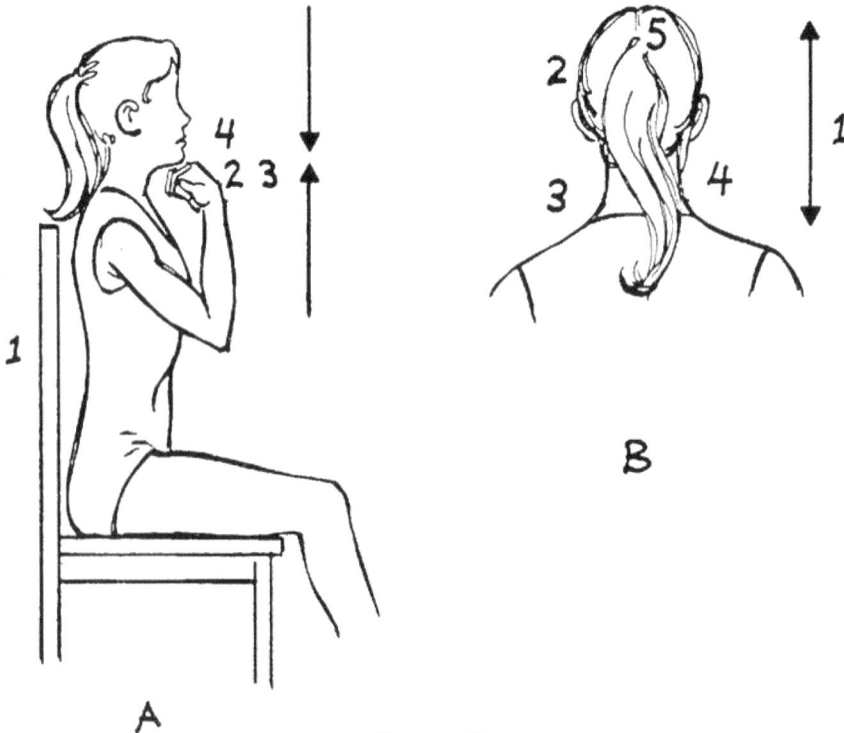

Figure 19
The Thoracev

to normal. The secret Yoga mov-asana to lift it is The Thoracev. Here is how to do it. (Follow Figure 19.)

The position to assume (Figure 19A)

1. Sit straight in a chair.
2. Close one fist and place it beneath your chin.

How to do this Yoga mov-asana

3. Push up gently with your fist. But
4. Resist with your chin. (Maintain your chin in a *horizontal* position, in other words.)
5. Push up harder still with your closed fist. But resist it still more with your chin.
6. Relax and repeat.

Frequency: 2 repetitions. 3 times a week.

What The Thoracev does for you (Figure 19B).

1. With each succeeding repetition, your neck stretches more. Its muscles and ligaments stretch. Hence, its vertebrae separate farther and farther, and their joints regain their flexibility.
2. Improves the circulation of your neck and brain.
3. Reduces considerably the threat of arthritis of your neck.
4. Relieves the cramped, "painful" feeling in your neck.
5. Restores your natural memory power, your creativity, your power of concentration, and the even balance between the nervous systems that control your body functions and your circadian rhythms.

How Tom V.'s Neck Felt Limber Again

Tom V. was tormented by a disturbing "tight feeling" in his neck. Like most subchronic ailments, it pestered him when he least expected and ruined his efficiency at work and his social relationships. Repeated medical diagnoses revealed nothing pathological. Still, something "pulled" at Tom's head and stiffened his neck, "like arthritis."

I taught Tom The Thoracev. Before he had repeated the prescribed two repetitions twice the first week, his head felt clearer (from the improved circulation), and the stiff feeling of "coming arthritis" vanished.

His neck soon felt amazingly flexible. His "lost" memory was fully regained, too, and his efficiency increased so remarkably that his superiors urged him to return to school at night and get a higher degree for an important promotion.

How to Protect Your Heart for a Long Life

To remain young enough to live a long life, you have, primarily, to care for your heart. This is especially true as you get older. While the Yogis (and I, too) vigorously oppose reminding people of their ages, you are perpetually being asked for it by professional men, institutions, the government, and other groups. Your heart rate, for example, says Fox,[6] is the key to determining how strenuously you ought to exercise, and your peak heart rate declines with age. Fox advises that, if you are forty and engage in light jogging or play doubles in tennis, don't let your pulse rate exceed 150 per minute.

The Yogis and I agree only partially with him. For over 25 years I have taught that you should forget that you are getting old as the guide to the speed of your heart rate. I have taught that you ought to build up your muscles instead and exercise as vigorously as you feel. All of us will die eventually, either while resting or while active. If your coronary (heart) blood vessels are not blocked and you suffer from no measurable heart deficiency, the worst that can happen to you if you over-exercise *by yourself* (not over-drive yourself in competition) is that you will feel tired and stop. No scientist has yet disproved my long-held (and Yogi-held) premise.

Scientists, though, wisely point out important precautions to take for your heart. Changes in weather, rather than the temperature itself, *can* affect your heart seriously.[12] Such changes impose unusual stress on your circulation, either by raising or lowering your blood pressure sharply. If your heart is deficient you will find normal breathing difficult in cold weather because the cold constricts the blood vessels near your skin and overloads your heart with too much blood to pump normally. It is, as a consequence, very important *not* to exercise outdoors in very cold or very warm weather unless your heart is unusually healthy. That is one sure way to protect your heart for a long life.

A Mystic Secret to Oust Lower Back Rheumatism (Lumbago)

The most likely cause of your non-pathological lower back

rheumatism (lumbago) is your exposing your lower back to a draft. You can catch one from outdoor sports when the.exertion warms you up, and you aren't clad appropriately to resist the physiological effects of a chilly wind. Jogging or bicycling for a considerable distance with a cold wind at your back could cause it. The larger your back muscles, the more you suffer because more muscle tissue will be "inflamed." People who "never" exercise are seldom afflicted with lumbago.

The condition may cause great pain and rigidity, making it practically impossible for you to move, to get up after you lie down, to walk, to sit down, and to get up again. Indeed, you can hardly move your bowels, for you suffer excruciatingly when your anal sphincter muscle contracts to perform the act, for it is attached to the string of the little bones of your lower back (your coccyx). You are crippled for the most common moves; in fact, for you can barely turn at the waist. Your back feels as if broken or crippled with arthritis. When your lumbago is established without doubt, this is the scientific Yoga mov-asana to follow:

1. Lie down on your side (preferably on your bed). Place a wet, hot towel (or more conveniently, a thermo-bag, or something similar) across the lower two-thirds of your back.

2. If you prefer, fill a bathtub halfway with water as hot as you can stand without burning yourself. Sit in the tub and recline against one end of it, using a thick, folded towel as a pillow.

3. Keep the hot water running slowly to maintain the water hot enough.

4. Remain immersed for about ten minutes, no more.

5. After the first few minutes in the tub, your rigid back will feel more limber. Whereupon, bend your body forward repeatedly in the tub to loosen the rheumatic tendinous attachments of your back muscles (especially those of your lower back). As your body gets warmer and more limber, bend forward farther and farther.

6. Then step out of the bathtub. If you also have a shower, turn it on as hot as you can stand without burning yourself, bend over halfway and let the water pour down over your back.

7. After one minute or so under the hot shower, bend down repeatedly as far as you can to stretch the inflamed tendons still more.

8. If you are staying home that day, repeat Numbers 1-7 four different times during the day. At the end of each time you will be more limber than the last and suffer less pain.

9. When you arise next day, the pain and stiffness in your back will feel as if they have returned in full! But don warm clothes and do The Yoga Back Curl, page 19. It will limber you up again and will remove the pain from your back

muscles. Take no more hot baths after that. They draw too much required salt out of your system.

10. Repeat the Yoga Back Curl (page 19) at bedtime. Repeat it again next morning upon arising. Your lower back rheumatism will be ousted. If a trace of it lingers on, repeat the Yoga Back Curl mov-asana that night and again next morning.

Important: Once you catch lumbago, it tends to recur at about the same time every year in the same muscles. If you don't oust it without delay it will spread through your back, into your shoulders and neck, and incapacitate you with excruciating pain when you so much as breathe! So, don't wait a day when it strikes.

Why Yoga Is So Effective with Sport Injuries

Although your injuries from sports and athletics may usually be the least immediately pathologically dangerous, they are usually the most painful. Such injuries range all the way from the simple "soreness" which you feel the day after a new exercise or after overdoing an old exercise, to cramps, sprains, inflammation of your joints (like synovitis and bursitis), traumatic inflammation of the tendons of your lower back muscles (lumbago), inflammation of your muscle fibers (fibrositis), the crippling stiffness following the overstretching of a group of your muscles, and so forth. When you make the least move, such extensive, nerve-filled anatomical areas flash great volleys of pain sensations to your brain, and you feel as if the world is coming to an end.

But the "bark" is worse than the "bite." And yet, you cannot ignore the pain, or it spreads or turns chronic. Cigarettes, in contrast, could be giving you lung cancer for years *without* causing pain. So, don't let the pain of a simlple athletic injury scare you away from exercising again later. Find easily, in the index , the specific Yoga secret instructions or mov-asana which rids you of it, and you will soon be exercising again.

The Yogi Method to Overcome Tennis Elbow

Regular indulgence in tennis, push-ups, golf, bowling, baseball, handball, and other arm-using sports and occupations tend to overuse and weaken your elbows. The resulting condition is commonly called "tennis elbow." It is chronic and painful when your arm is used. Your most used elbow is usually affected first, compelling you to favor it and overuse the other one—and strain it, too! Although the dictionary describes the misery as "a strain of the elbow with soreness of the muscles of the forearm," it feels more like an arthritis of the elbow joint. Your elbow may turn so tender that you can hardly touch it. When it is "tennis" elbow and nothing else:

1. Heat applications alone are little help, or the help might take too many months.

2. Rest your arm, *but only from the particular movement* which brings pain. Stop doing, for a while, in other words, *the particular* tennis stroke or movement in *the* sport or effort which brought on the condition. Even discontinue playing tennis (or the sport directly responsible for the pain) for a month, or two or three. Practice, though, the arm movements which cause *no pain*. Still use the affected joint and muscles around it, in brief, in movements that *don't aggravate* the condition, but which circulates fresh, nourishing blood through them which also removes their accumulated waste products.

Here is the Yoga mov-asana for it. (Follow Figure 20.)

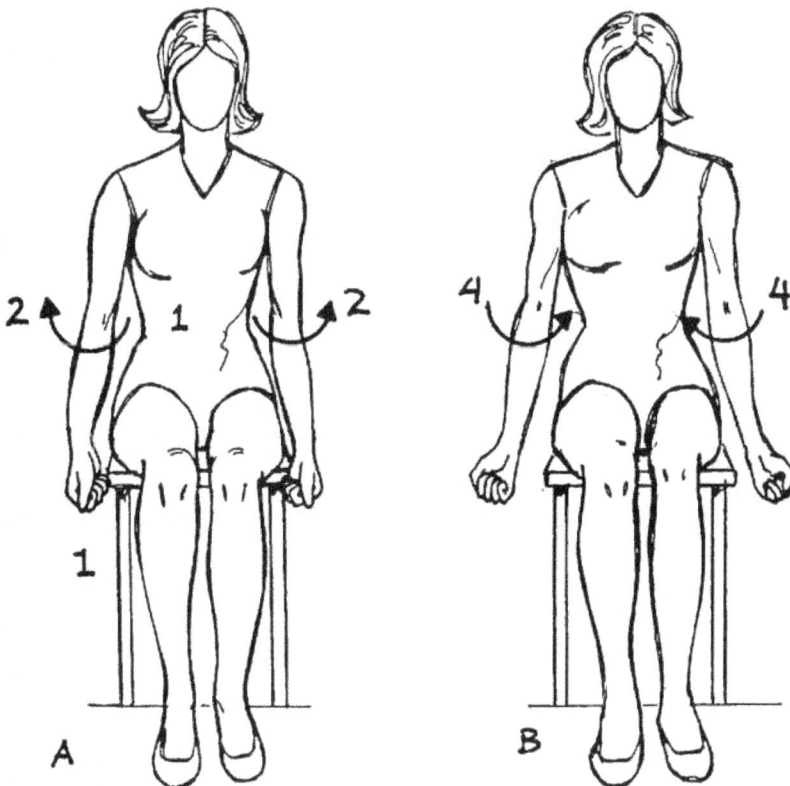

Figure 20
For Tennis Elbow

The position to assume (Figure 20A)

1. Stand or sit with your arms hanging loosely by your sides.
2. Close your fists.
3. Now, twist your arms *outwards*.

Frequency: Do it from 10 to 50 times. (Then Figure 20B.)

4. Repeat by twisting your arms *inwards* the same number of times.

What this Yoga mov-asana does for you:

1. Stretches the tightened, inflamed muscle attachments around your af-flicted elbow and reduces the amount of accumulated waste products in it.

Final words:

1. Repeat this arm-twisting mov-asana several different times a day. You can't remove the soreness from your muscle tendons by stretching them only now and then. You have to stretch them at *several different times* during the day. Even then, they will stiffen up again when you rest overnight. But they will limber up faster next day when you stretch them again.

2. In two or three days the tightened muscles will be stretched out again, the inflammation will diminish tremendously or vanish, and the crippling sore-ness will end. Otherwise, you could suffer from the malady for months or years, and from recurrences the moment you repeat regularly the original movement that caused it.

References

[1]Other medical centers, among the great many engaged in such research, are the Harvard Medical School, the University of California at Los Angeles, 14 universities involved with the Defense Department in five-year studies of mentally-controlled hand-warming techniques for soldiers working in cold cli-mates, and others.

[2]Frank Rudolph Young, *Solar Diet*, 1954, p. 22.

[3]*Ibid.*, pp. 6, 47.

[4]*Ibid.*, pp. 18, 27.

[5]*Ibid.*, p. 20.

[6]*Ibid.*, p. 22.

[7]*Ibid.*, p. 23.

⁸*Ibid.*, p. 23.

⁹Frank Rudolph Young, *Yoga For Men Only* (West Nyack, N.Y.: Parker Publishing Company, Inc., 1969).

¹⁰Dr. Jay D. Coffman, Boston University Medical Center. Scientific session of the American Heart Association.

¹¹Dr. Samuel M. Fox III, President-elect of the American College of Cardiology. At a meeting of Chicago doctors.

¹²Frank Rudolph Young, *Cyclomancy: The Secret of Psychic Power Control* (West Nyack, N.Y.: Parker Publishing Company, Inc., 1966), p. 56.

6

How Yoga Allows You
to Maintain Your Vitality
Through the Years

How a Secret Yogi Alpha Brain Wave Changes Your Outlook

Most people are somewhat afraid of growing less attractive as they grow older. The threat frightens you early in life, grows with the years, and turns your natural, healthy brain waves wild. Since *all* your brain waves are projected *from* your brain into your body, your physiology responds to their inharmonious rhythms, your facial expression may turn "sour," and you may come down with mysterious ills. Use *your own natural brain waves* to discipline these discordant brain waves to restore your health and sweeten your expression. The scientific Yoga mov-asana to achieve this is Your Face-Sweetening Alpha Brain Wave. Here is how to do it.

1. Sit or lie quietly (later you can do it standing) and let every care be banished from your mind. Shirk off even the most pressing ones, if you can do so safely.

2. Close your eyes at first to do this simple mov-asana more easily.

3. Don't try to feel drowsy, as in the true alpha state. Feel, instead, alive, eager, and super-attractive. Stop thinking, nevertheless, and "feel" ready to participate in the most thrilling, "senseless," *un*inhibited behaviour. But you will still retain the power to control yourself, for you are *not* in the true alpha state.

4. Flood your whole body with this "feeling." Feel it rush from your brain into your body and permeate your every cell, from head to foot. And let your glands (your thyroids in your lower neck and your sex glands in your loins)

saturate your whole system.

5. Your expression will sweeten, as if by magic.

How to expand your outlook into a conquering one with this mov-asana

6. Let this "feeling" pour out of you from every direction and float out to people and enclose them like a delightful warm fog.

7. Visualize the warm fog settling into their tissues. "Feel" the fog spread through them, right up to their brains. "Feel" it adapt itself to the vibrations of their own brain waves and to alter them into the vibrations of *yours*. Visualize this strongly enough as if it is happening, and it *will* happen.

8. Practice this Yoga secret several times, and you will be able to do it instantaneously with people.

9. You will be so amazingly irresistable to others that your whole outlook will change, You will become attractive to those around you, and not feel "abandoned by the human race."

How Margaret W. Threw off Her "Poisoning" Mind

Margaret W. suffered from "mysterious" ills which defied diagnosis. She told me that she found life increasingly unbearable. No matter how much she strained herself to please others, nobody seemed to appreciate her. People just wanted still more from her and took further advantage of her. It baffled Margaret because she was not unattractive. But she saw life passing her by in an endless chain of lost dreams. And yet, she was a conscientious person and went out of her way to please others! She just never felt "really well" anymore.

I asked Margaret to stare suddenly at herself in the mirror. She agreed that she did look rather stern. "But I have always looked like that!" she explained.

"That's why I think you are having these strange troubles," I replied. The grave slant of her expression detracted from her sexual and social appeals and drove people from her. People's reactions confused and frightened her, and her natural, healthy alpha brain waves turned erratic. Their resulting inharmonious rhythms *could* victimize her with mysterious ills which her physicians found undiagnosable.

Margaret practiced Her Face-Sweetening Alpha Brain Wave. It

flooded her whole body with the feeling of being intensely alive, eager, and super-attractive. Then she stopped thinking, as directed, and "felt" ready to participate in the most thrilling, "senseless," uninhibited behavior. But she retained the power to control herself!

Her "mysterious" ailments vanished as if by magic. Her expression sweetened, and she suddenly looked much younger and prettier. People sought her now for *herself*. She no longer had to "kill herself" to please them. Her mind stopped "poisoning" her.

How the Yoga Mystic Cyclone Works

The tortures of your conscious thinking overwork your mind with excessive apprehension over insignificant threats to your future, be it in security or romance. Your brain, as a result, is forced to replenish its energy constantly with new supplies of pure blood loaded with its main

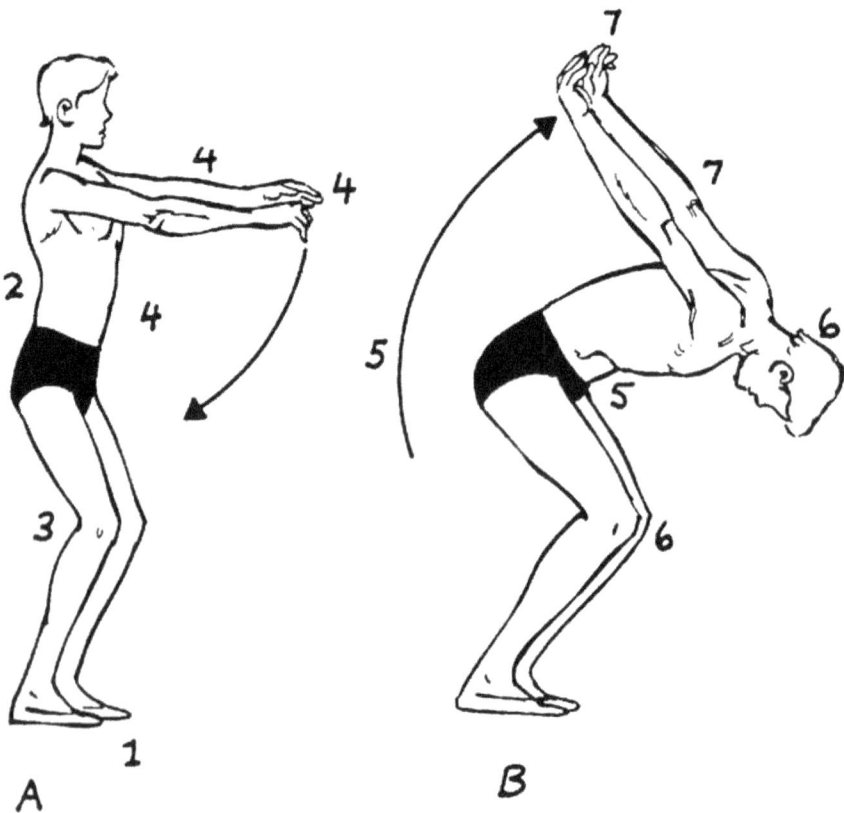

Figure 21
The Yoga Mystic Cyclone

food, oxygen. The excessive apprehension overflows into your subconscious mind and saps your energy even more when you sleep. Hence, you cannot build up a reservoir of energy, and you feel tired even after resting. The simple Yoga mov-asana to overcome this energy-destroyer in you is The Yoga Mystic Cyclone. This is how to do it. (Follow Figure 21.)

The position to assume (Figure 21A)

1. Stand with heels normally apart (from 10 to 14 inches), depending on your height, toes pointing normally slightly outwards.
2. Hold your back straight.
3. Bend knees slightly.
4. Inhale and raise arms straight out, palms down.

How to do this Yoga mov-asana (Figure 21B)

5. Exhale and swing arms backwards. At the same time,
6. Bend forwards, and bend knees much more.
7. Swing arms way back and up, palms *still* down.
8. Repeat without pause.

Frequency: 10 repetitions. 2 sets (groups of repetitions). 5 times a week.

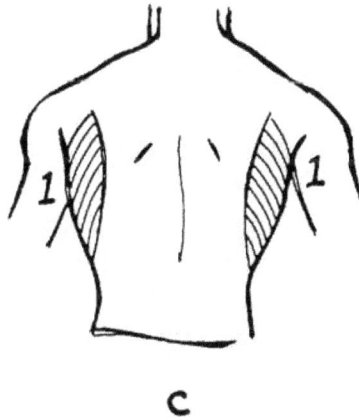

C

Figure 21, cont.

What the Yoga Mystic Cyclone does for you (Figure 21C)

1. Proportions your outer upper back.

2. Stimulates your whole circulation, triggering your adrenal glands into secreting more dynamic hormones.

3. Thus, it fills you with energy and better prepares you to meet the outer world because it toughens you to some of its ecological unpleasantness.

How to cement this necessary state into you all day long:

4. It alters your natural brain wave into one which protects you against the unavoidable onslaughts of the world you live in. Now,

5. Aware yourself keenly of how you feel when in it. Then practice assuming this feeling at will several minutes afterwards. If you don't succeed at first, repeat the mov-asana about four times to get the right ''feel.''

6. Assume this brain-wave state thereafter at work, when shopping, or doing anything ''upsetting.'' Assume it so completely that your brain radiates into you the brain waves which protect *you* against the world. Reassume it repeatedly during the day and keep filling yourself with energy.

How Eddie K. Learned to Breeze Through His Long, Dreary Work Days

Eddie K.'s daily work left him feeling listless, lackadaisical, and fatigued. He awoke in the morning so supersensitive to sound, taste, and smell that he complained about everything. All day long, everything went ''wrong'' with him. Nothing pleased him. Everybody else was ''idiotic.'' He hadn't a friend in the world.

Since Eddie was diagnosed by his own doctor as being organically sound, I knew his problem was his outlook. The tortures of his conscious thinking were apparently overflowing into his subconscious mind and sapping his energy, even when he slept.

I taught Eddie the Mystic Cyclone of Yoga. With the Mystic Cyclone Eddie altered his own natural brain wave into one which fortified him against the onslaughts of the world he lived in. Thereafter he assumed that brain-wave state at work, while shopping, or doing anything ''upsetting.''

His conscious thinking lost its torture and he conserved his energy. He was soon breezing through his long, dreary work days.

How to Stop Wasting Your Physical Currents

A leading European doctor agrees with the Yogis that too much ambition can make a man impotent.[1] Worrying about careers ruins the sex lives of an increasing number of young men. It causes them to ignore physical exercise, to feel always under a strain, and to develop a fear of failure in their jobs or a fear of sexual impotence. Their wives may be partially responsible for their plight, too, by pushing them to get ahead in their careers.

If you are overly-ambitious, you are also prone to heart attacks and stomach ulcers. Such over-ambition uses up your nerve-electricity excessively and reduces your natural physical voltage—and your sex energy. Sex stimulation fails to stir you enough thereafter, for your sex glands turn less responsive. Their brain centers are repressed by your over-seriousness and by the abnormal demands of your mind and body for energy to carry out your ambitions. The urge to indulge in sex play and other romantic activities diminishes, and you turn into an abstaining aesthetic. It might drive your marriage on the rocks.

To avoid this peril, refuse attractive career offers if they will overtax you. Seek work that lets you operate, as much as possible, at a satisfactory pace without feeling as if being rushed. Then flow along with that pace.

After work, exercise from 45 minutes to an hour. Select the Yoga mov-asanas which you enjoy most, and do them eagerly and feel your muscles bulge (if you are a man), or then beautify you (if you are a woman). By concentrating on doing them correctly you take your mind off your work and enjoy again the delights of your home and the thrilling intimacies it provides you with your mate. Such reflections will restore your natural physical voltage at any age, and you will enjoy life as you go along, instead of postponing it for a future date that might never come.

How the Air You Keep in Affects Your Energy Level

No matter how deeply you exhale, a considerable amount of air still remains in your lungs. This is the air you "keep in." When more of this air is "bad air" (carbon dioxide) your energy level is low. When too much of it is "good air" (oxygen) you feel faint because your breathing slows down. When this air consists of the right amount of good and bad air, your heart beats normally at its best pace, you feel at your strongest and possess your most energy endurance. The effective Yoga mov-asana to put the best air mixture into the depths of your lungs and keep you going at your best for hours is Your Energy Feedback. This is how to do it. (Follow Figure 22.)

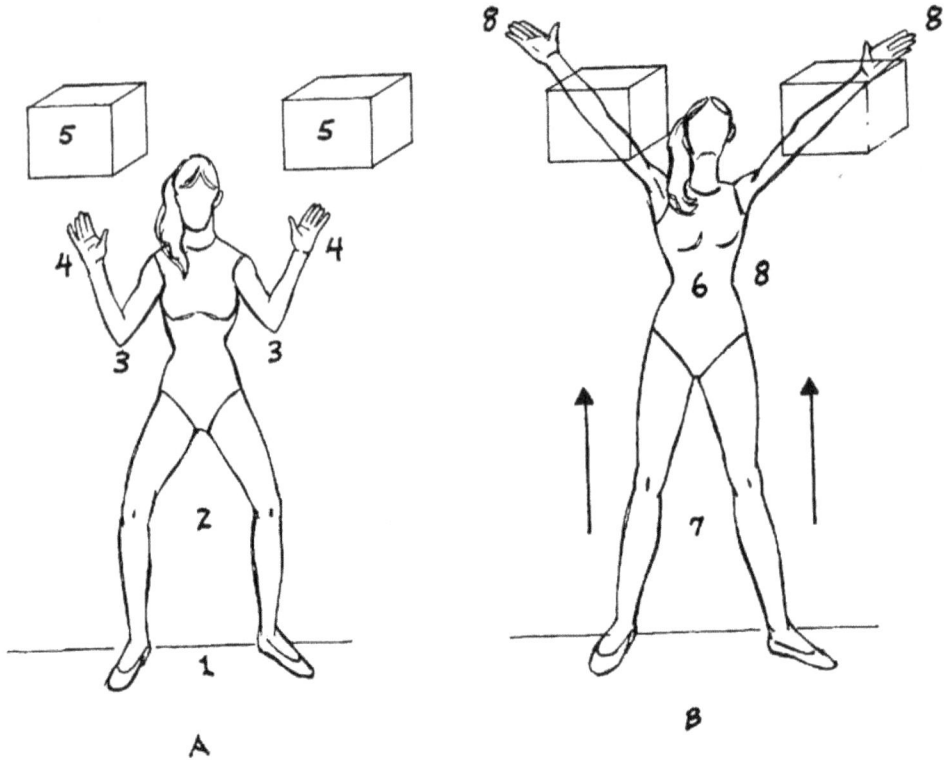

Figure 22
Your Energy Feedback

The position to assume (Figure 22A)

1. Stand with feet comfortably apart. Set your heels from 10 to 14 inches from each other, and your toes pointing normally slightly outwards.

2. Bend your knees slightly, to about one-fourth down.

3. Keep your elbows against your sides, but

4. Place your hands, palms forwards, close to your shoulders.

5. Imagine that the obstacles you are encountering that day are walling you in the air around you.

How to do this Yoga mov-asana (Figure 22B)

6. Inhale deeply. Then

7. Straighten your knees fast. At the same time,

8. Exhale, and thrust your arms straight out in a direction midway between your head and your shoulders (or at a 45 degree angle to your body).

9. Do so with vim. Visualize your arms as two powerful spears which rip through your obstacles (the wall-like air).

Frequency: 10 times. One set (group of repetitions) a day.

What the Energy Feedback Mov-asana does for you:

1. Slenderizes your waist.

2. Stirs up your circulation.

3. Flushes the "bad" air out of your lungs and normalizes the air mixture deep in your lungs. You are put at your best energy level, and it feeds it back into your whole body. Your mind seethes with original ideas.

4. Tones up your heart and your thighs.

5. Stretches your spine.

How Ames C. Blew off His Body Poisons Every Day

Ames C. had turned into an utterly discouraged person. He was sick and tired of fighting obstacles. He lost his appetite and no longer cared what happened to him. Psychiatrists and other counsellors and personality schools urged him to make friends. But he made only enemies. Although he was found to be organically sound, he didn't feel "like himself" in anything he did. He made little headway with women, too, even though he was physically attractive.

I taught Ames the Energy Feedback mov-asana. Next day, already, he sensed a delightful "tuning" in his head. It left him feeling so free and contented that he made more friends that very day, socially and in business, than he had made any other day in his life. Waves of zest for life from his lungs seem to ripple all through him. Even when he strolled through crowds he felt these "waves of life" burst out of him and put people around him under his domination. He regained his appetite and dove into the stream of life as if born again.

Effect of the Yoga Bent-Over Press on Your Arteries

To lower your blood pressure when it is high, or to raise it when it is low, you have to alter your physiological rhythm through your sympathetic nervous system. Your splanchnic (visceral) blood vessels are the storehouse for your surplus blood. When you tighten your abdominal muscles, you draw more blood to them *from* your splanchnic blood vessels, and your blood pressure rises. After you relax and rest your abdominal muscles, your blood pressure falls again. This is the up-and-down effect on your blood pressure which the Bent-Over Press has. By mastering this effect on your physiological (circadian) rhythm with your mind, you can control your blood pressure at will *anywhere*. This is how to do the Bent-Over Press Yoga mov-asana. (Follow Figure 23.)

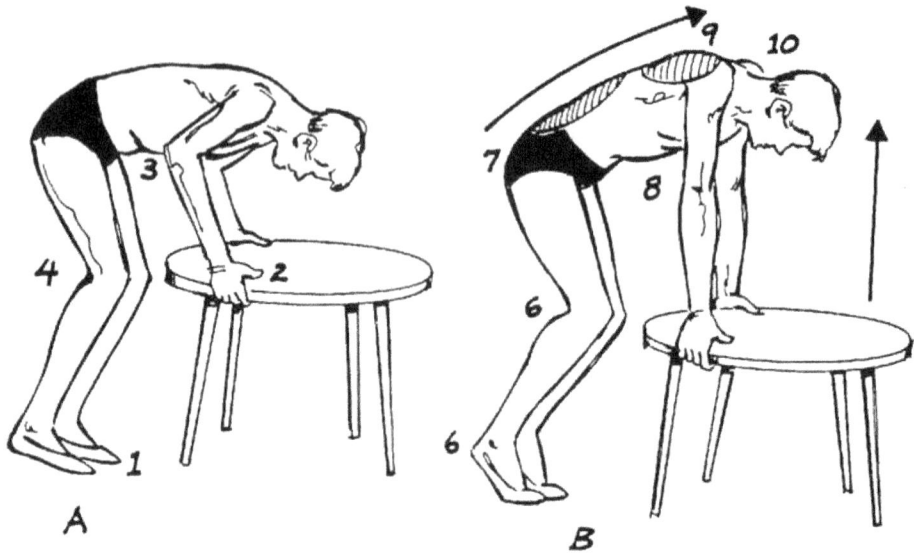

Figure 23
The Bent-Over Press

The position to assume (Figure 23A)

1. Stand close to a round stool.
2. Rest heels of hands (palms down) on edge of stool.
3. Bend elbows, but keep them parallel to each other.
4. Bend knees and lean body far over stool, as if you are falling over it.

How to do this Yoga mov-asana (Figure 23B)

5. Do numbers 6,7,8,9, and 10 *all at the same time*:
6. Bend knees more, and go up on toes.
7. Draw in hips.
8. Straighten arms, and
9. Round your back still more.
10. Round your shoulders.

11. Tighten chest and abdominal muscles at the same time.

Frequency: 4 repetitions. 4 sets (groups of repetitions). 3 times a week. Do any set with any one of the 3 grips described below.

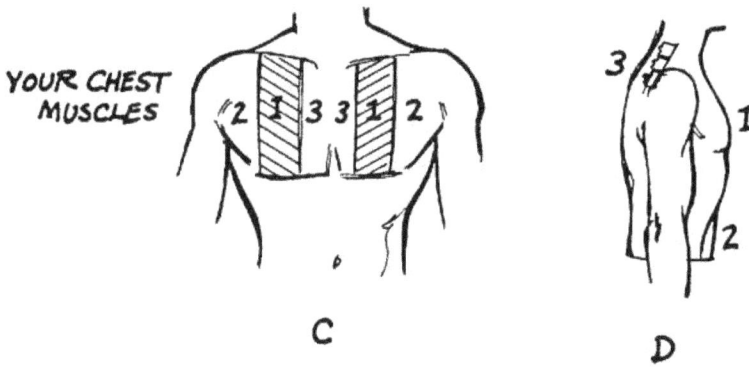

Figure 23, cont.

What the different grips do for you (Figure 23C)

1. Normal grip (hands placed shoulder-width apart) rounds out the middle section of your chest.

2. Wide grip (hands placed 2 inches outside shoulders) rounds out outer sections of your chest.

3. Close grip (hands placed nearly 2 inches within shoulders) fills out the inner portions of your chest.

4. Moving your body slightly forward when straightening it, in addition, fills out your whole chest.

What the Bent-Over Press mov-asana does for you (Figure 23D)

1. Unsurpassed as a chest muscle or breast stand-upper. Your chest muscles or breasts feel as if being drawn right off your body, so fast do they enlarge.

2. Your abdominal muscles contract so tightly that they shrink your waist unbelievably. You burst with confidence in your abilities.

3. Stimulates the vertebrae of your upper back (your 3-4-5 dorsals) to improve the functions of your liver, diaphragm, lungs.

How to lower your blood pressure with the Bent-Over Press

1. After each of the first two sets sit down and relax your abdominal muscles thoroughly by leaning forwards, with your elbows resting on your thighs. Your splanchnic blood vessels will follow suit reflexly and relax and store up your surplus blood again, lowering your blood pressure.

2. Grow keenly aware of how different your abdominal muscles feel in that position from when they are tight while engaged in the Bent-Over Press.

3. After each of the two last sets *sit straight*. Your abdominal muscles are *not* thoroughly relaxed then. But think them into feeling *as relaxed as they were* when you leaned your elbows forward on your thighs. Think them into relaxing thoroughly all the way down from your ribs to your hips. Your splanchnic blood vessels will respond reflexly to your thinking, relax, and will store up your surplus blood again and lower your blood pressure.

4. With a little practice you can reproduce that same "thinking mood" any time you wish, anywhere, and your blood pressure will be under your control. (*Note*: If your blood pressure problem is pathological, see your doctor or other healer).

How Robert N. and His Wife Commanded Their Blood Pressures

Robert N. suffered from a steadily-rising blood pressure. His wife's was rising, too, but less fast. As a precaution Robert arranged to partially retire from his job, but his blood pressure did not fall enough to warrant his sacrifice in pay and style of living. He had heard of brain wave devices for training the lowering of blood pressure, but had little confidence in equipment attached to his head and preferred a more "natural" means.

I showed Robert N. the Bent-Over Press, and he asked me to teach him this simple movement. He enjoyed it at once, for it made his chest muscles enlarge with incredible speed. He enjoyed still more sitting down after each set and relaxing his abdominal muscles, first by resting forward on his thighs, and then by merely thinking himself relaxing. His physiological rhythms synchronized, and he said that he could actually "feel" his blood pressure lowering.

With a little practice Robert could reproduce that same "thinking mood" anytime he wished, anywhere. He soon felt more limber, he said, and knew that his blood pressure had "gone down." His chest muscles, meanwhile, enlarged so remarkably that his wife, Aimee, tried the same simple Yoga mov-asana to increase the size of her breasts. Robert told me her breasts "bloomed like mushrooms."

Aimee added the "blood pressure thinking" to her exercise and learned to control her blood pressure, too. Robert and Aimee lost their fears of developing uncontrolled blood pressures, and that alone multiplied their power of command over the threatening condition.

How a Yogi Refreshes His Body with Every Breath

No matter how strong or sturdy you think you are, without sound lungs you cannot expect to live long, nor to be healthy to the end. People with barrel chests, in fact, are frequently subject to lung ailments.

Yogis have always believed in *exercise* for lung disease. Western doctors, in contrast, have prescribed quiet and rest to save the strength of the pulmonary patient. My medical ancestors in the miasmatic tropics agreed with the Yogis instead and with their secrets cured many a lung patient. Science at last agrees with their methods. Lung disease patients are now being asked to jump onto exercise bicycles, walk the treadmills, and do step-up tests. Exercise, the modern researchers have found, is particularly important for people with "smoker's diseases," such as bronchitis and emphysema, for asthma, and for people recovering from pneumonia.

But there is a problem. When lung patients exercise, the resulting forced deep breathing hurts their chests and makes them cough. That's why they won't exercise willingly nor do deep breathing exercises. They grow weaker, as a result, and develop new health troubles, like insomnia. Then they exercise still less, using insomnia as a further excuse for inactivity.

The Yogis totally disregard the natural pain in their chests when they exercise violently or deep breathe for their lungs. The forced deep breathing of exercise expands their lung space, especially at the upper ends, near the neck, where it is most liable to tuberculosis because it is aereated so little. Forced deep breathing resulting from violent exercise *aerates* this part of the lungs and starts it back on the road to health. That's why a typical Yogi can expand his chest from four to *seven* inches. Such an expansion potential protects him against lung trouble, no matter how much he exposes himself to the worst elements. For such chest expansion, do the Solar Breath mov-asana (see p. 17).

The Extra Yoga Secret to Refresh You

In addition, for any lung ailment eat garlic twice a day with heavy meals. The garlic fumes pass from your blood into the air-spaces in your lungs, attack the bacteria in them, and dry up the infectious mucous and the inflamed mucous membranes. This makes more lung space available for breathing and brings back lung health.

Warning: Don't sit or stand straight when you cough. If you have a lung or throat illness, no matter how slight, bend forward at the waist when you cough, at right angles to your legs. Dislodge the mucous plugs in your lungs with the least trauma to their mucous membranes. Then dispose of the mucous where it cannot dry and spread through the air and recontaminate you and infect others—perhaps even your loved ones.

If you experience lung trouble after exercising violently, try to rest by lying down from one-half to one hour after the exercising to let your body regain its used-up energy quickly.

With garlic every now and then, and with the Solar Health movasana, you, too, can refresh your body with every breath.

Avoiding Loss of Your Inborn Energy Supply

A recent health article read, "Too Much Exercise Can Kill You, a Doctor Warns."[2] Since childhood I have heard such frightening words. Around 1910 or so, the world's best-known strong man was the German "blond Adonis," Eugene Sandow. He died suddenly of a heart attack in his early 50's just after performing a Herculean feat on the stage. The hue and cry went up that "exercise kills you young" by cursing you with an "athletic heart." Textbooks poured out upholding the new dogma, and the public grew terrified of physical exertion.

The "warning" doctor of the aforementioned article approved of moderate and regular exercise, however, agreeing that it could improve remarkably the efficiency of your heart. Excessive physical exercise, though, which makes your heart work too hard or fast, he cautioned, should be avoided. I myself have *dis*believed that precaution all my life. I have exercised vigorously repeatedly over the years, even though I've had many intervals of enforced idleness to study or recover from many sport injuries. And I am in fine health. I have also taught my exercise system to others since 1947 to people from 10 years old to 94 years old, at a time when the world still considered "exercise" a life-shortening "dirty" word.

A study, however, at last supports my lifetime practice and teachings. "Vigorous exercise can prevent heart attacks," a British research group finds.[3] It will help prevent heart attacks regardless of the age of the person, and *even* if he smokes! Lighter exercise does not offer a comparable protection!

I was right, then, as far back as my childhood. My lifetime results and teachings uphold it. I do agree with the "caution" doctor, however, on one point. It is unwise to enter physical contests or games as a way to build up your health. The safest and most lasting gains in health and body building, I have always insisted, whether you are a man or a woman, are made by *exercising by yourself*. You *force* yourself when you play games—you *compete* with your muscles—to equal or surpass someone else's achievements. That is a dangerous physical practice, and psychologically, it is traumatic. You no longer aim primarily then to build up your health and perfect your body so much as to outclass another person in skill, muscle power, and reflex speed. Such a goal has little to do with sound health or body symmetry, but to incline you to overstrain. You strive to perfect *the* athletic skill during practice and risk suffering from such chronic ailments as tennis elbow, lower back arthritis, torn tendons or ligaments, synovitis of the knees, bursitis, hernia, slipped disc, sprain after sprain, fallen arches, varicose veins, or even broken bones.

When you exercise by yourself, though, or even with someone else without trying to better him (such as, when you and your mate do the same Yoga mov-asanas), you concentrate on doing them *sensibly and correctly*, exerting yourself only as much as you wish to. You don't labor under the nervous tension of trying to "beat" a rival, or of being beaten and "humbled" by him (or her). You can halt your workout anytime you wish without being "riled" for it and being called "getting old." You will not waste your inborn energy supply and drive yourself to energy suicide.

When you do compete in a game, however, do so for the fun of it. Expect to lose when you are not at your best to win, and congratulate the winner wholeheartedly. Should *you* win, of course, feel happy about it. But don't subject yourself to the tension of the "potential winner," or you will take dangerous chances, as Eugene Sandow did, and strain yourself by attempting physical feats which are beyond your capacity at the time.[4]

How to Feel Always Raring to Go

Your volcanic emotions waste, in spurts, an incredible amount of your energy. They can saturate your body with wastes, or flood the blood vessels of your head with blood and give you a pounding headache. They can drain blood from your alimentary tract and leave you suffering from indigestion, constipation, and other visceral ills. Your temporarily over-stimulated sympathetic nervous system can deplete your energy. Protect yourself against its depleting effects by feeling always raring to go. The Yoga mov-asana for that is Your Yoga Energy Depot. Here is how to do it. (Follow Figure 24.)

The position to assume (Figure 24A)

    1. Lie flat on your back, legs extended normally.

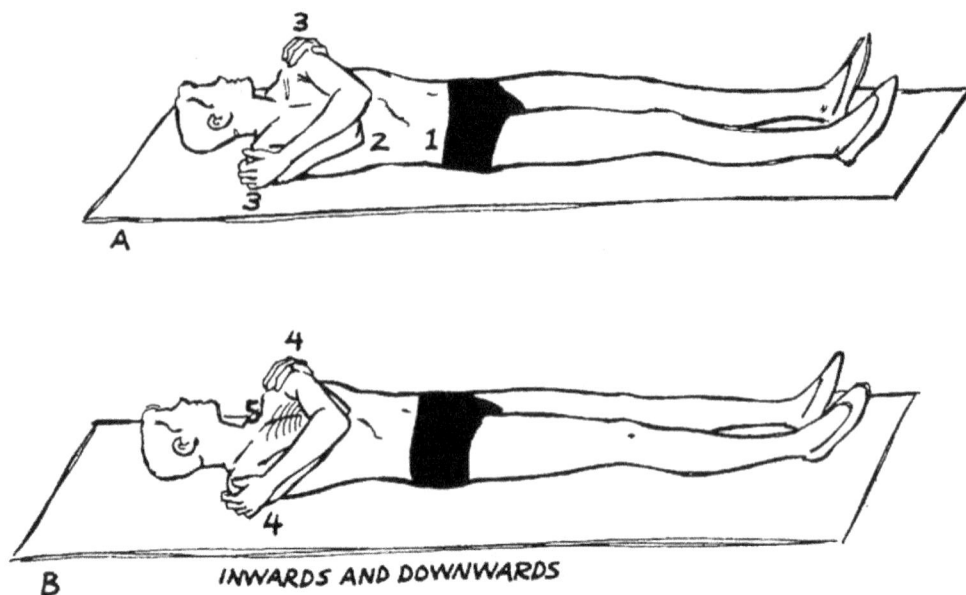

Figure 24
Your Energy Depot

2. Cross arms over your chest, with left elbow resting on right elbow.

3. Cup left shoulder with right hand, and right shoulder with left hand.

How to do this Yoga mov-asana (Figure 24B)

4. Press shoulders inwards and downwards with hands. At the same time,

5. Firm your chest muscles hard. Feel the inner groove of your chest bulge tightly.

6. Hold the firming (or the contraction) for two seconds.

7. Relax and repeat. Each time you firm the groove with each succeeding repetition, you will feel more energy collect in it.

8. By the time you reach eight repetitions, you will feel so much energy collected in that groove from your adrenal glands that your whole chest will throb with it.

9. You will then have trapped superhuman energy within you and will feel raring to go.

Frequency: 8 repetitions. 1 set (group of repetitions). 4-5 times a week.

What Your Energy Depot does for you (Figure 24C)

1. Enlarges amazingly the inner thirds of your chest or breasts.

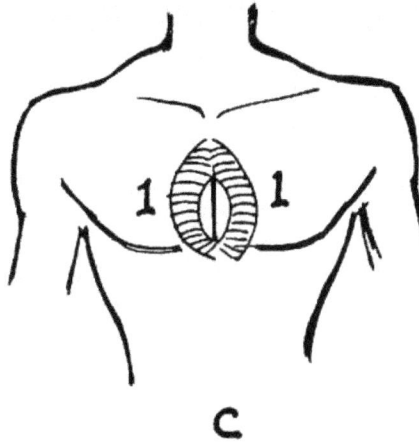

Figure 24, cont.

2. These muscles are among the bulkiest muscles of your body, so when they feel full, you feel bursting with energy.

3. Your adrenal glands are excited thereby, both by these muscles and your mind. These muscle-toned muscles have turned into energy depots, and you feel raring to go. Socially and in business you will be a leader.

How Larry K. Trapped Super-Vitality Within Him

At 55 Larry K. was utterly discouraged. He felt that youth had passed him by, he feared being assaulted and robbed by large, vagrant youths, and he didn't expect to live much longer. His employer seemed likely to let him go in a big cost-cutting program.

I told him that his life lacked worthy, controllable stress. "You live longer," I explained to him, "when you have something to passionately cling to, like a child, a loved one, a pet, a hobby, a career, a long-range plan, or some other gripping goal."

I taught Larry His Energy Depot. He felt it enlarge the inner thirds of his chest muscles amazingly. Since they were among the bulkiest muscles of his body, the bigger they felt, the more energy he felt bursting within him.

Larry determined to make himself so strong that he would stop being afraid of his own shadow. He practiced His Energy Depot for two months and built up enormous chest muscles. In an unexpected predicament he performed a feat of strength that equalled that of a professional strong man's. The confidence in himself which he suddenly displayed at work urged his employer to appoint him to a higher position, instead of laying him off.

Larry had another gripping passion now: the passion to live long and still remain unusually strong. He is near 80 now, and is so daring and youthful that he swims out-of-doors in icy weather, belonging to the city's Polar Bear Club.

References

[1]Dr. Ernst Gaderman, Hamburg University, Hamburg, West Germany, 1973.

[2]Dr. Ray H. Rosenman, Department of Medicine, Zion Hospital Medical Center, San Francisco, California.

[3]London School of Hygiene and Tropical Medicine, London, England. (*Lancet*, leading British medical journal).

[4]More and more statistics uphold me. Jim Londos, the clean-living world wrestling champion for 16 years, who competed 30 years against thousands of opponents, died in 1975 at about 75-80. Top-seeded tennis player in 1933, and captain of the Davis Cup team in 1951, Francis X. Shields, died the same day at 64. Both men had died of heart attacks. Many more world-famous athletes have done little better. Competitive sport in itself is NOT the road to longevity.

7

How Yoga Helps You
Live a Long, Healthy Life

Daily Health Hazards and How to Combat Them

Some of the worst health hazards you face every day are:

1. *Noxious air pollutants*, like ozone and nitrogen oxide. They endanger the health of your lungs and may cause emphysema (the formation of trapped pockets of air in your lungs). The best safeguard against these pollutants would be to live where they don't exist. Since that is virtually impossible or impractical nowadays, a vitamin E-rich diet, for the most part, has been found to protect your lungs from them.[1] Once your lungs are damaged, though, no amount of vitamin E can help to restore them to their previous state.

The Yogis derive their vitamin E from foods. It is present in large amounts in green lettuce leaves, cottonseed oil, corn oil, peanut oil,[2] and wheat germ oil, but not in olive oil. It is also found in meat, butter, milk, eggs, and fish liver oils. Rancid fats destroy it by oxidation.

The Yogis, though, do not get their vitamin E from concentrated oils. Lettuce twice a day, I insist, contains all the vitamin E you need. I myself take no stand for or against concentrated, bottled oils, but, like the Yogis, I resort *only* to the natural sources for any food or medicine. The nutritional content is unquestionably reduced during transportation and storage, but that is nothing new with man's food. Even the villagers transport their produce from farm to market, to be sold the day after it is picked. It remains out of cold storage all that time, and on the way to town it is exposed to the scalding rays of the sun, which seriously diminish the vitamin content of most foods.

In colder climes, where people live longer, foods picked in the summer and fall are stored in basements and eaten all winter. That has gone on for thousands of years. You would have to live on your farm and eat your food the moment you pick it, like the birds and animals do, in order to extract the utmost vitamin content from it. Yet, for centuries people *not* on farms have lived long lives! Right in a super-polluted city like Chicago there are dozens of centennarians who have lived in it their whole lives! So, it is still possible to get your daily necessary vitamins from foods in stores, provided that you don't ruin the food afterwards with overcooking, over-exposure to light and heat, and so on. You also have to select the freshest foods you can.

2. *The weather*. Scientists finally admit that the weather can have disastrous effects on your health. Heart attacks are more common when the weather is extremely hot or cold. During periods of bad weather, far more emotional disturbances take place. The majority of suicides in America are committed when it is either snowing, raining, or overcast. Your nerve-electricity is reduced at such times. The carbon monoxide in the air is also increased, threatening you with more accidents on the road because breathing carbon monoxide makes you less alert—or stupefies you. You are even more subject to nose bleeds when the sulphur dioxide level in the atmosphere is above average. Watch yourself on such "wrong" days and protect yourself.

Yoga Secrets to Block the Path to Cancer

If you drink liquor you face a greater risk of getting cancer of the mouth, warns Dr. Robert Lindley, chief radiologist at the M. C. Anderson Hospital and Tumor Institute in Houston, Texas. No wonder the Yogis don't drink!

The Yogis knew how to prevent cancer of the bowel. They ate foods which, worldwide studies have shown, were not consumed by people who developed bowel cancer. These foods possess a high fiber content.[3] Fibers are that portion of your food not digested by acids in your stomach. They hasten the passage of your food through your colon, thereby preventing it from stagnating in it, as occurs when you eat "soft" foods, processed foods, and other foods with little bulk content.[4] The high fiber content effect, many scientists believe, permits minimal contact of the cancer-producing agent present in your diet, with the lining of your bowel.

But I don't think that this is the major reason why such foods help to prevent cancer of your bowel. I believe that since your food fiber (the bulk in your food) holds water, it keeps your fecal matter moist and porous and far less resistant to the onward pushing of your peristaltic wave than the comparatively dry, hard, solid fecal matter created by "soft" foods. Such pliable fecal matter does not bruise, blister, and rip the lining of your colon, as does the hard, slowly pushed along fecal matter. It spares your colon from such a repeated trauma and from the resulting overgrowth (hypertrophy) in spots which can end up in cancer. In beef-eating countries, like Denmark, Scotland, Argentina, Uruguay, and the United States, the incidence of bowel cancer is rising fast because meat lacks the water-holding fiber (bulk) necessary to create more porous, more moist fecal matter. So, eat foods with bulk to block the path to cancer.

A Miracle Toner for Your Brain and Upper Body

Your brain and body have to be in balance with each other if you hope to live a long, healthy life. Only then will your physiological (circadian) rhythms synchronize with each other and enable your body to function at its long-living best. Otherwise, your physiological rhythms are thrown out of focus with each other and you fall victim to an unexplained tension, fatigue, and other malfunctions which throw your system out of order and overburden your heart. Your upper body carries the key to overcoming this threat to your longevity because it contains your vital organs. It also houses, in your spine, the nerve connections between your body and your brain. Tone up your upper body and it will flash toning-up voltages to your brain. These will, in turn, balance your brain with your body and automatically synchronize your circadian rhythms for a long and healthy life. The secret Yoga mov-asana for this miracle is The Yoga Palms Down Press. Here is how to do it. (Follow Figure 25.)

The position to asume (Figure 25A)

1. Stand backwards against your kitchen sink; or something equally firm, and no higher.
2. Set your palms near the edge of it, with
3. Fingers pointing outwards, sideways. Wear protective gloves.
4. Space your hands less than shoulder-width apart.
5. Bend knees a little, and drop your body by several inches.

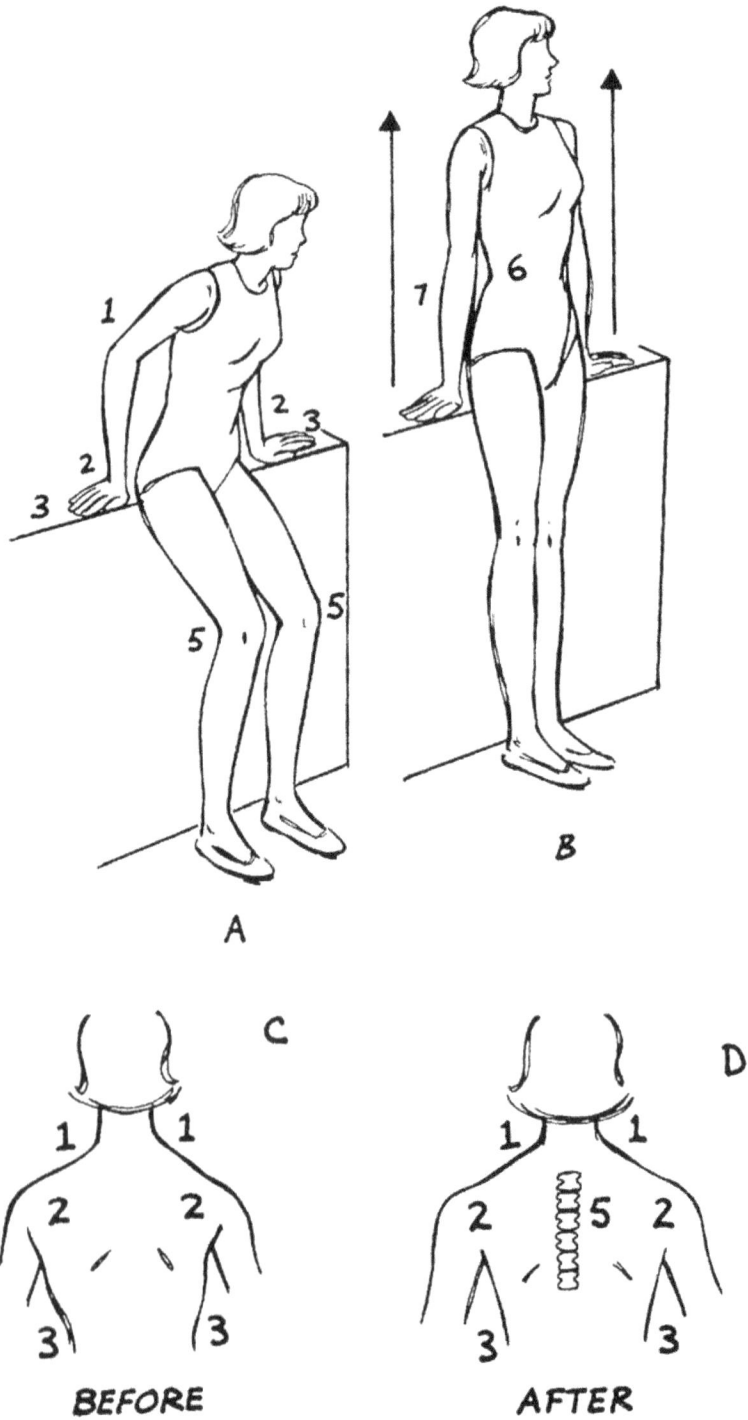

Figure 25
The Yoga Palms Down Press

How to do this Yoga mov-asana (Figure 25B)

6. Now inhale and arch your back.

7. Straighten your arms, raising the weight of your body. Try to bring your shoulder blades together, if you are a man, for upper middle back.

8. Repeat.

Frequency: 6-8 repetitions. 2 or 3 sets. (groups of repetitions). 3-4 times a week.

The Yoga Palms Press (Figures 25C,D—examine both sides)

1. Glamorizes the first section of your trapezius muscles, which hold up your shoulders and combats round shoulders.

2. Glamorizes your posterior deltoids, which keep your shoulders back, and help keep your back straight by reminding your subconscious mind of its posture.

3. Glamorizes your inner triceps, which firm and shape your inner arms.

4. Is very important in helping and healing bursitis of the shoulders, as well as arthritis and subluxations of the back.

5. Triggers your three cervical plexuses of nerve because it separates enough of the first four vertebrae in your upper back, immediately below your neck, to stimulate the nerves that pass through between them. That tones up your head and face, neck, heart, and lungs. Alerts your brain.

How Lucia Q. Kicked Age off Her Back

Lucia Q. suffered from a tired upper back at the end of her day. She noted, in time, that she was feeling shorter. Indeed, she even looked shorter than before when standing next to people she knew for years. Her defect was postural, but it would lead to arthritis of her neck, to a permanently bent upper back and its resulting compression of the spinal nerves to her heart, lungs, and stomach, and reduce their blood circulation. Her circadian rhythms would be thrown out of focus and decidedly shorten her life.

I taught Lucia the Palms Down Press. When she dropped her body by several inches to do it, she felt her upper back stretch straighter. It was a unique and welcome sensation. Her shoulders were forced upwards and backwards at the same time, automatically strengthening their muscles and holding her back up thereafter without her conscious control.

Next day she suffered less at work from a tired back. In a surprisingly short time her upper back was much straighter, and she looked taller and more elegant. The base of her neck no longer nagged her with discomfort. She felt 20 years younger than before. Her mind cleared.

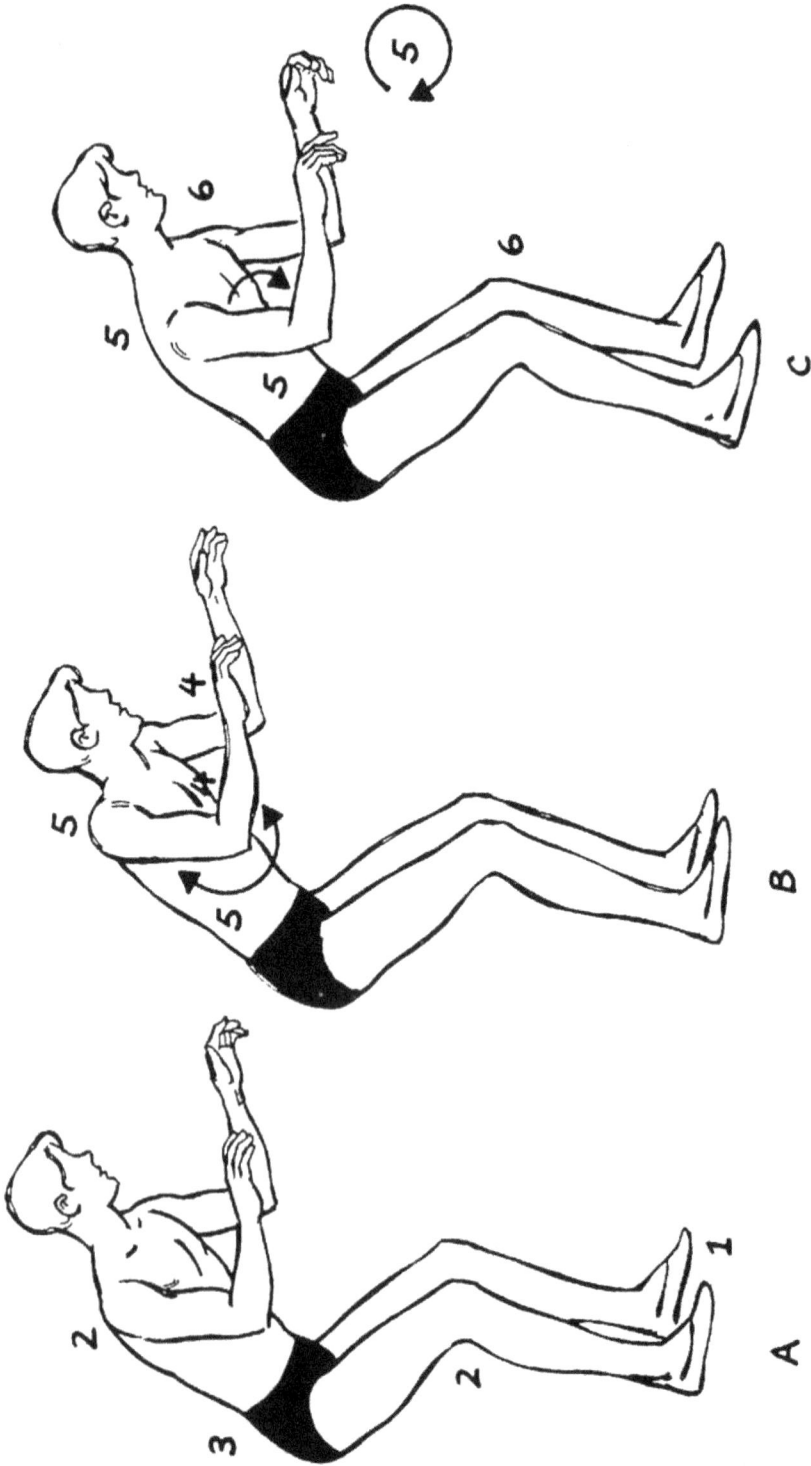

Figure 26
Your Shoulder Rock and Swing

The Secret Yoga Mov-asana to Resist Disease

The Clutch of Gravity on you continuously lowers your resistance to disease (no matter if the malady is infectious or chronic, or resulting from the wear-and-tear over the years). That's why you ought to include brief periods of rest during the day. Otherwise, by overfatiguing you, the Clutch of Gravity adds lactic acid, urea, and other waste products to your blood and weakens your resistance to disease. It is important for you to know how to counteract this ruinous fatigue. To enjoy stable good health, you have to follow *regular* habits. (The Yogis discovered this thousands of years ago, and the Russians now also believe it.) I myself revealed, in detail, those secrets of constant good health and long life 20 years before the Russian[5] (and now the American) scientists discovered them.[6] In addition, I found that you must also regularly prevent The Clutch of Gravity from weakening you noticeably during your waking hours and disturbing your physiological (circadian) rhythms. An example of this weakening when you travel is "jet fatigue." It severely breaks down your resistance to disease. The Yoga mov-asana to counteract it greatly is Your Shoulder Rock and Swing. Here is how to do it. (Follow Figure 26.)

The position to assume (Figure 26A)

1. Stand with heels from ten to 14 inches apart, depending on your height, toes pointing normally slightly outwards.
2. Bend knees and crouch forwards,
3. But keep your back rather straight. (That is, don't slump forwards.)

How to do this Yoga mov-asana (Figures 26B,C)

4. Keep elbows at sides, and bend them at right angles to your body.
5. Rotate shoulders by swinging elbows in circles while keeping forearms nearly at right angles to the floor.
6. Throw your whole body into the "rock and swing." Let your trunk and knees fall into the swing. (Figure 26C)
7. Do this stimulating Yoga mov-asana with energy and glee.

Frequency: 10 circles (repetitions) of your elbows. 3 sets (groups of circles.) 5 times a week.

What Your Shoulder Rock and Swing does for you:

1. Fills you with ecstasy and synchronizes your various circadian rhythms with each other.

2. Renders your shoulder joints more flexible, greatly preventing bursitis.

3. Stimulates circulation in your arms, legs, back, and chest.

4. Counteracts fatigue and increases resistance to disease. Improves health substantially. Fills sluggish shoulders and back with feeling of glee.

How Vilma K. Felt Ill No More

Vilma K. was tired of getting sick easily. It cost her many hours of pay, social appointments, and the respect of friends and acquaintances. She seldom looked her best, and seldom felt fit. She was always recuperating from something, it seemed, for she was always catching one thing after another.

Since she was not pathologically ill, I assumed that she was suffering from a daily ruinous fatigue that markedly reduced her natural resistance to common ailments. I informed her, first of all, that the Yogis, like the Russians, have found that to enjoy stable health she had to follow *regular habits*. Secondly, she had to prevent the Clutch of Gravity on her from weakening her noticeably during her waking hours and disturbing her circadian rhythms.

So I taught her The Shoulder Rock-and-Swing mov-asana. It filled her with ecstasy and synchronized her various circadian rhythms with each other. Her sluggish shoulders and back suddenly felt flexible. Her arms, legs, back and breast came alive with racing blood. Vilma's fatigue left her day after day. Her natural resistance to disease zoomed, and she was soon living like a normal, healthy person again.

How to Chase Sickness Away

Investigator Ring[7] discovered, following extensive tests, that many diseases were firmly linked to specific emotions. For thousands of years the Yogis have insisted that all diseases can be cured with the mind. Christian Science has upheld them. Indeed, so has every religion. Among such diseases, which even the investigator confirmed, are: gallstones, heart disease, diabetes, migraine headaches, colitis, peptic ulcer, arthritis, asthma, high blood pressure, ulcerative colitis, and even tuberculosis.

There are many diseases, though, which are *not* necessarily caused by specific emotions. Take, for instance, arthritis from overuse of the neck in carrying heavy loads. Village women in India (and Central America) are subject to it from toting large containers of water or of produce to the city market on their heads. The pain or discomfort, or both, engendered by such a disease can convert you into an apprehensive sufferer or worrier who overreacts to fear. Your sympethetic nervous system then turns super-reactive, leaving you prone to ulcers and heart attacks.

If you are the type who fears ridicule, you conceal your fear and anger deep within you and can suffer, as a result, from skin diseases, colitis, and worsening arthritis.

If you are the type who reacts tempestuously to diseases, you may suffer from asthma, diabetes, high blood pressure, and migraine headaches. In other words, you *invite* these diseases.

To stop inviting disease, follow a carefully worked out health program. But once you *are* ill, strive *calmly* to get well again, or you will invite *other* diseases and turn sicker still. Realize that, ordinarily, you won't get well overnight from a malady that took years to develop in you. There is too much in your system to repair or correct. The healing process can't be hastened, except by a miracle. But neither can you neglect the illness. You may have to alter many of your daily habits for some time. You may have to do a number of specific Yoga mov-asanas for it. But do them all, and do them *confidently*—and improve day by day. Suddenly, you will feel "like yourself" again. That is how to chase illness away.

Three Secret Yogi Musts to Stay Healthy and Live Long

The Yogis have long followed three secret musts to stay healthy and live long. These are:

1. *Long distance running*. It lowers your cholesterol level, enlarges your lungs to breathe in more fresh air with each breath, lowers your blood pressure and slows down your normal pulse rate. No marathon runner of any age has been found with fatal coronary diseases (Basler).[8]

But I disagree with Basler's claim that those who jog for short distances still die of heart attack. And I feel eminently qualified to say so. My medical and Yogi ancestors and I ran for exercise most of our lives. For decades I was ridiculed for it. Until the late 1960's I was stopped in three big American cities and questioned by the police for running in the parks after dark. So, I doubt if anyone has been more watchful of the lifetime effects of running on the body than I.

From the private tests which I have conducted on others and myself on two continents, one in a tropical and the other in a cold climate, I conclude that short sprints, interrupted by brisk walks ranging from one to three times the distance of the sprints, also lowers your cholesterol level, enlarges the volume of your lungs, and lowers your blood pressure. I haven't found it lowers the pulse rate, but neither do I consider that alteration a necessity for a long life. Such a lowering might even be *un*natural. Paavo Nurmi, the famous, unbeatable Finnish Olympic runner and world record holder in the middle distances in the 1920's, trained in long distances to develop the endurance with which to win in the middle distances (5,000 meters, or nearly three miles). Yet, he died in his early 70's of a heart attack. I am convinced that his pulse had slowed, too, as it does with runners of the marathons. On the other hand, there are people who live to 80, 90, and older with *normal* pulse rates of 71-72.

A slowed pulse (of 40 to 50 beats per minute) suggests to me symptoms of bradycardia (a too-slow heart), similar to the dangerous condition brought on by anesthesia. Like my ancestors, I insist that a normal heartbeat, particularly one between 70 and 72 beats per minute, is the ideal. I cannot agree with the widely-held scientific premise that a heart has a "pre-ordained" number of beats before it stops beating, and that the slower it beats the longer it will last. I insist (and science, I predict, will eventually prove me again to be right) that, barring physical and physiological accidents, your heart muscle will beat as long as it remains sound and your coronary arteries and heart valves function normally. The number of beats (contractions of your heart muscle), I declare outright, are no more subject to a "pre-ordained" number than your biceps muscle is subject to the number of contractions it can make in your lifetime before becoming useless. I'll say the same for your heart's pacemaker, which triggers it to beat. Your pacemaker should be able to stimulate your heart to beat so long as the cells that comprise it remain healthy, no matter how many times it has stimulated it before. Your pacemaker, otherwise, will eventually stop stimulating your heart muscle when its cells surrender to pathology or old age, and not because it has stimulated your heart to its "full quota" of contractions.

Hence, I repeat, a healthy heart that beats comparatively slowly has no better chance of beating for a longer time than a healthy heart that beats at the normal pace of 70 per minute or so. If your heart beats too fast, of course, there is a danger that its muscle will hypertrophy (enlarge abnormally) from the over-activity and bring on the coronary pathology of the "athlete's" heart. But its shorter "life" will be due to the over-development of its muscle, not to its faster beating. This is one more of my scores of far-ahead-of-my-time prophecies for which I expect to be universally-upheld eventually. So, I advise you that in order to stay healthy and live long, prefer short sprinting with intermittent brisk walking to long jogging. It will, besides, traumatize your knee and hip joints far less because you will take less steps even if stronger steps.

2. *Do not plunge into icy water*, unless you are used to it. Swimming powerfully in cold water (as far down as 56° F.) after warming up with exercise on land, makes you vigorous, resistant to colds, builds up tremendous energy, and develops a strong heart. People in colder climates, it has been proved repeatedly, live longer than those in warm climates. Swimming in water colder than 54° F., though, (unless you are accustomed to it, like the bravest Yogis and the long-lived people of the Caucasus Mountains) might be risky. "Icy" cold water (50° F. or less) slows down the flow of blood through the leg veins and is thought to be a major cause of clots.[9] Such clots can cause phlebitis (an inflammation of the veins of the legs), and even death if the clots travel through your bloodstream and lodge in your lungs. The Yogis prepare themselves to endure extraordinary cold. To be healthy, though, it is *not* necessary for you to join them in such a feat.

3. *Avoid heavy drinking*. It is wisest, in fact, to drink no alcoholic beverage whatsoever. Heavy drinking, according to Missouri University psychiatrists, makes you allergic to most foods.[10] Such an abnormal allergy prevents you from eating nutritious foods and dooms you to a shorter and, sooner or later, unhealthy life.

Social drinking, too, raises the level of fats in your blood. It has long been known that heavy drinking affected the liver, heart, and coronary (heart) blood vessels, but studies show that even social drinking can harm the same parts of your body.

Secrets to Retard Aging

As your body grows old, more and more of its muscle cells turn to fat—or "die," so to speak. More and more elastic fibers "die" in your face and let it wrinkle. More die in your arteries and deprive them of the power to contract, converting them into blood-containing pipes instead of actively-pumping blood vessels. These inevitable changes lead to your final death. The Western world accepts these alterations in you as scientific facts and resigns itself to them.

The Yogi does not. With sheer force of mind he *blocks* such alterations—or their speed of occurrence—by *refusing* to accept them. . . by *refusing* to accept the fact that he is growing older every day. . . by *visualizing* himself as remaining *always* at a selected age, say 28, *no matter how old he grows*. He *does not* taper down or soften the rigors of his life. This powerful mental attitude, the Yogi has proved, retards the "inevitable" changes of his cells with age. With this unshakeable belief that his *mind* governs the age of his body, he commands his body, with his mind, *never* to grow old—and his body responds to it to an astounding degree.

Your Secret Ideal Age to Keep You Young

This is how to apply this Yoga secret. Pick an ideal age for yourself which you would always like to remain. (Say, 28, because at that age you are considerably matured mentally and have reached your physical peak.) If you reached your peak earlier, pick *that* age instead. If you reached your mental peak at 35, and your physical peak at 24, then visualize your mind remaining the rest of your life at 35, and your body at 24. If your mind is still maturing and improving at 54, but your body passed its peak at 23, then visualize your mind remaining at 54, and your body at 23. Pick whatever mental and physical ages you would like to remain all your life. See yourself thereafter as remaining *that* age (or ages), and live as if your mind and body *were* those ages. Ignore your birthdays from the standpoint of chronological age. Celebrate them if you choose to, but forget the number of years they indicate on your birth certificate. Then continue visualizing—and acting—*as if you were still* the ideal age (or ages) mentally and physically which you have picked for yourself.

Visualize this ideal age (or ages) so vividly and so constantly that you practically hypnotize your mind and body *to return to*, or *to remain*, that age (or ages). Such repeated thinking flashes commands continuously from your mind to every cell of your body and *converts them* into the kinds of cells which you visualize them to be, just as the mind of the miracle self-healer converts his sick cells into healthy cells.

Don't, for one moment, let that ideal health picture of yourself slip out of your mind—even when you consider your true age in official forms. Let the number of your actual age become, to you, *just another number*. But let the picture of yourself at your ideal age become, to you, *an actual reality*. When you stare into the mirror thereafter, see yourself always at your ideal age (or ages). When you participate in sports, do likewise. Naturally, compete only when fit, or you could strain yourself *at any age*. But don't fill yourself with defeat beforehand because of your acquired negative attitude towards your chronological age. Yet, don't drive yourself in the competition until you are exhausted, either! You can always compete again another day. So, in anything you do, always visualize yourself as remaining at the ideal age, mentally and physically, that you wish. Like the Yogis, you *will* retard old age and live a much longer, youthful life. Start doing that *right now*.

The Natural, Pill-less, Yoga-like Diets of Two Incomparable World Champion Athletes

Herb Elliott was an Australian who engaged in sedentary work. He broke the mile record in the 1950's in 3:54.5. (Three minutes, fifty-four and a half seconds). His record stood for years. Very much like the Yogis, he trained on oats, nuts, raisins, dried fruit, and diced bananas. For practice he ran 20 to 40 miles a day, barefoot, in the Australian bush country. He swam and wrestled before a big race and didn't even warm up for the race in standard style. Yet, so fresh did he finish his races that he went an extra lap at a speedy clip to receive the plaudits of the crowd. Then he immediately spoke over the loudspeaker system. Had his competition been stiffer, he would have broken his own record repeatedly. Herb Elliott was a slender, bookwormish, white-collar worker in his 20's who ran wearing spectacles.

Another spectacular athlete of the late 1950's, and who is still one in the middle 1970's, is Eder Jofre. He is a Brazilian around 40 who also trains on a Yoga-like diet. As a youth, he won the bantamweight boxing championship of the world and retired undefeated after a seven year reign. Years later he returned to the ring and fought his way up to the featherweight title. He is still undefeated. All during his career Jofre has punched like a heavyweight and moved like a flyweight. He fights the full 15 rounds, too, when the bout goes the limit, without being exhausted. He is wealthy, possesses a movie actor's figure, looks like an Adonis, and boxes like a master swordsman. He wastes no blows, seldom gets hit, and lands lightning thunderbolts himself.

Both Herb Elliott and Eder Jofre testify to the effectiveness of a Yoga-like diet for speed, power, endurance, wonderful body proportions, and long-lasting competitive bodies. So stop being misled by the theory that a Yoga-like diet is a debilitating one. It is not a heft building one, but it cannot be surpassed for giving you health, power, agility, and longevity.

Foods to Strengthen Your Heart (Four Secret Rules)

Yoga food secrets to help your heart, if it is afflicted, are widely-accepted in Europe and South America. My medical ancestors were the first to use and spread this knowledge in the Caribbean and Latin America. Use it yourself without waiting for America to accept it. Here it is:

1. Eat an abundance of fresh citrus fruits, bananas, figs, potatoes, tomatoes, and other foods with high potassium content.

2. Avoid foods which contain salt. Examples of such foods are: ham, cheese, seafood, celery, beets, spinach, eggwhite, sausage, most breads, beer, nuts, and packaged, canned, and bottled fruits. (The last contain sodium benzoate, a salt preservative.) Salt compels your heart to work harder to pump your blood through you, overburdening it. Also avoid diuretic (urine-triggering) drugs. They cause your heart cells to lose potassium, a chemical essential for your heart's function.

3. In brief, if your heart is not up to par, follow a low-salt, high potassium diet. The premise is that salt is harmful to your heart-muscle fibers, while potassium *protects* those fibers. Salt, you see, attracts water to your heart muscle-fibers and overburdens them.

4. Vitamin C also helps to remove cholesterol from your body, thus preventing the building up of fat deposits in your blood vessels. Such deposits contribute to heart attacks. According to Ginter, of Czechoslovakia, vitamin C helps enzymes in your liver remove cholesterol from your body.[11] That's why a vitamin C deficiency can lead to eventual heart attack.

Caution: As stated on page 47, an *excess* of vitamin C can increase your chances of a heart attack. So, I recommend, unless your doctor or professioal healer orders to the contrary, confine yourself to natural sources of the vitamin.

The natural sources of vitamin C are citrus fruits (oranges, grapefruits), canteloupes, strawberries, potatoes, fresh peas, asparagus, and lettuce. Other sources are cabbage, turnips, tomatoes, and spinach. But since the last group of food is usually cooked, they lose considerable amounts of their vitamin C. This vitamin can be taken in capsule form; but then you deprive yourself of the roughage in the food originally containing it. Bran and other roughage is commonly added in its place, but, like the Yogis, I contend that Nature intends you to consume each vitamin in its natural milieu, rather than extracted and concentrated or eaten with an alien roughage added to it.

How to Protect Your Heart for a Long, Healthy Life (Ten Secrets)

Newspaper editors and reporters constantly face deadline pressure and intense competition. They lead the top of the Friedman list of heart attack-prone occupations.[12] I myself have written prolifically for over 40 years, and have published (myself and by others) for 25 years. I have been subjected to that pressure since my late teens. Yet my heart is in perfect shape. Why? Because I learned early the Yoga secret to protect my heart for a long, healthy life. Here it is, revealed at last. Let it do for you what it has done for me.

1. When in the heat of a "rush" to do anything, say to yourself, "trying to go too fast makes me go too slow. I make too many errors then, and waste too much time correcting them. So I'll take my time NOW, no matter what! I'll make sure I don't have to retrace *one single step*. I will still keep my word and complete my duty—but in *my own* best way."

2. Then, think ahead as you proceed, *one step at a time. Don't try* to combine different steps for a "short-cut."

3. But don't *overspend* time on any one step. If you are short for time, leave out any step or two that you can't do satisfactorily. Do nothing half-well!

4. Waste little time arguing, disputing, backbiting, or "battling mentally" with people who irritate you. Always deal with them good-naturedly, and turn "immune" to their insults.

5. Do some strong exercise every day. Sprint at top speed several times, from 20 to 100 yards, depending upon your running condition. Between the sprints, walk from 2 to 4 times their lengths. (Or a total of four mov-asanas.)

6. Then sit down and do three sets of Your Rude Awakener mov-asana (page 203). It will tone up your back muscles and turn you strong and confident to meet—and overcome—any obstacles. It will also prevent you from tiring easily from the constant pulldown of gravity on your neck and shoulders.

7. To feel strong enough to carry the world on your shoulders, like the pagan god Atlas, do The Torso Push (page 36-38).

8. End up with the Myotatic Toner (page 27) to ease the compression of your spine by the downpull of gravity, on the spinal nerves which stimulate your heart. You thereby allow your heart to regain more normal blood circulation in a *natural manner* and to increase its strength and normalize the power of its beat.

9. Lie down and rest for a half hour before supper to divide up your day. You will be refreshed in body and mind for the rest of the evening. If you could rest, too, before lunch, even for much less time, so much the better. It is not necessary for you to fall asleep during these rests, although that does not hurt. But you should stretch out, preferably with your head no higher than your body.

10. If you are heart attack prone, you will greatly minimize, if not completely halt, the tendency.

That is how to protect your heart for a long, healthy life.

Foods Believed to Add at Least Ten Years to Your Life

Without knowing the scientific reasons why, Yogis have, for a long time, favored foods which scientists prove now contain a large amount of antioxidants. Antioxidants inhibit oxidation and thus prevent "aging." The best diet for such foods comes from a vegetable rather than a meat source. You yourself can procure such foods in polyunsaturated margarine, eggs, vitamin C (oranges, pineapples, tomatoes, red peppers) and wheat. Walker, in experiments with rats, found that large doses of antioxidants increased their lifespan 12 to 14 percent. In a human being that would amount to about ten years.[13] Since the Yogis and my medical and dental ancestors and I never have, and never will, encourage you to take large or concentrated doses of any particular food substance, we recommend you to eat antioxidant foods regularly and avoid the possible side-effects and unpredictable long term effects of the untried. Increase your life-span safely! Don't take the chance which the takers of steroids and other body-building drugs do, as I warned body-builders 20 years before the scientific proofs supporting it were available!

A Yogi Secret to Live to 140, or Much Older

Despite all their self-imposed discomforts, a considerable number of Yogis have lived extraordinarily long lives. It is difficult for strangers to learn their longevity secrets because they keep so much to themselves. Having descended from a long line of them, however, I am no stranger to these secrets.

Science, at long last, is beginning to agree with these secrets. An eminent medical man finally predicts that people, like you, will live to 140 years. The Yogis predicted that for centuries. Many of them have lived much longer. One of their primary secrets was to make their bodies practically immune to infection. Dr. Walford (UCLA) has found that your body's antibody mechanism, which normally defends you against infection, starts failing as you grow older. It also starts to work *against* you, and aging sets in.[14] To live long as you grow older you have to live more protected from infectious disease and from degeneration of your body cells.

The Yogi achieves that goal through eating, once a day if possible, germ-battling foods, like raw garlic. He also habitually exposes himself to rather chilly weather in order to increase his resistance to sudden weather changes. You yourself can't add raw garlic to your breakfast or supper regularly and still retain your job. But you can, and should, eat it at least once on weekends when you don't socialize much. Certainly eat it on weekends when you go camping, jogging, playing tennis, swimming, gardening, fishing—and skiing, if you can get away with it. If your friends ridicule you for its sulphuric odor, laugh back and tell them that you are protecting *them*, too. In any event, don't be upset if your outdoor friends criticize you for it, for they will tolerate it if they like you as a person. It will lengthen your life by a nice percentage.

Note: Despite what you hear, nothing you eat, like parsley, will eliminate the sulphuric odor of raw garlic. Garlic's life-lengthening fumes permeate your bloodstream and are exhaled by your lungs. They don't combine chemically with parsley.

Don't pamper yourself at home with a room temperature above 68° F. Don't overdress indoors, either. Don't open your windows wide during chilly or cold weather. Enough air seeps in through your windows when they are opened between two or three inches, or even less, depending on the wind and its direction. Opening your windows wide in cold weather, besides, even at night when you sleep, causes your face muscles to contract for hours on end to fight off the cold. Your face, by morning, will be a mass of wrinkles.

The Yogis and I, too, believe that you should exercise *no less*, if you possibly can, as you grow older. More and more of your muscles degenerate or turn to fat with the years, leaving your muscles naturally weaker. But by exercising your remaining functioning muscle cells *vigorously regularly* you maintain your total muscle capacity closer to your prime's and lose less of your physical energy. Your prospects of living much longer than otherwise are considerably enhanced, then.

The Secret "Biological Clock" to Live to 200

Many Yogis, as stated before, have lived to beyond 140. One, it is claimed, reached to 450. Others are said to have ranged in age up to 250. I have made these revelations in previous books. The Yogis have long insisted that practically *anybody* can live to 200. Science has laughed at them. It was just a matter, the Yogis declared, of slowing down the speed of your internal tissue life. My Yogi ancestors revealed to me the secret of how to achieve this miracle.

Science finally agrees with them. It agrees that you *can* set back your own "biological clock," as the scientists call it, and reverse your aging process and live to 200 (Drs. Comfort, Prehoda, Swarts, and others).[15]

Studies on the lifespan of fish and other lower animals reveal a 10 percent increase in their lifespan for every degree their body temperature is reduced. Hence, one scientist (Strehler) predicts that sleeping on cooled water beds could do likewise for humans and add 15 to 25 years to human life.[16] The scientists expect soon to be able to reach into the core of your body's cells and "reprogram" them for a longer life. But the Yogis have been doing that for centuries already and living extraordinarily long—and youthful—lives! How do they do it? It will be explained shortly.

One scientist found, first of all, that by reducing the caloric intake of mice he caused them to live much longer and to be free of tumors, too.[17] Another scientist, however, found that by feeding mice *saturated* fats instead of unsaturated fats, they lived 20 percent longer.[18] So, changing your food won't do it alone, although (despite the findings of the last scientist cited) eating *un*saturated fats should favor your possible longevity more than saturated because the *un*saturated forms plaques that narrow and clog your arteries. The unchallenged requisite, though, is to *slow down your biological clock and bring it rhythm regularity*. A *speeded-up* life process (a speeded-up physiological clock) *kills* innocent victims of progeria, or children who are old by the time they are 11 or 12, and people with hyperthyroidism.[19]

That is the secret of the Yogis. They *slow down* their biological clock and bring it rhythm regularity with Yoga mov-asanas, such as Your Resting Back Arch Fortifier (page 15), Solar Breath (page 17), doing them in a furious sprint to throw off their excessive calories, and letting their bodies cool down afterwards, and with the Torso Push (page 36-38) to release their excess sex energy. They also eat raw fruits and vegetables to lower their body temperatures. Shaving off your pubic hair lowers your body temperature still more (More about this in "How A Yoga Secret Stops Wasting Your Physical Voltage," page 179). So does a daily cool bath.

References

[1]Dr. Daniel B. Menzel, Duke University Medical Center researcher.

[2]Dr. Tze Chiang, Engineering Experiment Station of the Georgia Institute of Technology.

[3]Frank Rudolph Young, *Solar Diet* (West Nyack, N.Y.:Parker Publishing Company, Inc., 1954), p. 18.

[4]*Ibid*.

[5]*Ibid*., pp. 12-13.

[6]Dr. Igho No. Kornbluch, chief of the physical medicine department of Northeastern Hospital in Philadelphia, and a team of scientists, at a biometeorological conference in Philadelphia. (*Midnight*, March 5, 1973).

[7]Dr. Floyd O. Ring, from extensive tests at the University of Nebraska School of Medicine. (*Midnight*, March 26, 1973.)

[8]Dr. Thomas J. Bassler, in a report to the American Medical Joggers Association.

[9]Dr. Jay D. Coffman, Boston University Medical Center. Scientific session of the American Heart Association.

[10]Dr. George A. Ulett, Chairman of the University of Missouri psychiatry department, with a group of the university psychiatrists.

[11]Dr. Emil Ginter, Institute of Human Nutrition Research in Bratislava, Czechoslovakia. *Science*.

[12]Dr. Meyer Friedman, Director of cardiovascular research at Mount Zion Hospital in San Francisco, California.

[13]Dr. Ronald Walker, Surrey University's department of biochemistry in England.

[14]Dr. Roy Walford, University of California at Los Angeles, California.

[15]Dr. Alex Comfort, leading British specialist in studies of the aging.
A Rand Corporation study for the government predicted a 50-year increase in the average human life span by 1990 to 2023.
Dr. Frederick C. Swarts, Lansing, Michigan.
Dr. Robert W. Prehoda, scientist.

[16]Dr. Bernard Strehler, professor of biology at the University of Southern California's Rossmoor-Cortese Institute for the Study of Aging.

[17]Dr. Clive M. McCay, 1934.

[18]Source unknown.

[19]*Rhythm regularity* is the name I gave bio-rhythm when I published my discovery of it in *Solar Diet*, 1954, about 15 years or more before science discovered it.

8

How Yoga Enables You
to Command Emotions
With Extraordinary Effect

How a Strengthened Body Produces Emotional Power

Whether you are a man or a woman, when you are flabby, constipated, or suffer from a chronic ailment, you are but a shadow of your best
self. But when you feel firm all over, with your bowels fully evacuated
and have no "sore feelings" or pains anywhere, you turn intoxicated with
your feelings of well-being. You move with a spring in your step and
carry a natural, cheerful attitude which is infectious. It draws others to
you and puts them under your control without a crumb of effort on your
part. The total effect fills you with an unconquerable, irresistible emotional power. Your faults and drawbacks vanish in thin air, and you
achieve your goals without even trying. Tasks which seemed difficult to
perform before, become "easy as pie" now. Years of personality training
could not bring you one-fourth of the emotional power over others which
you suddenly acquire. The Yogis have known this for centuries. That's
why they perform miracles without even trying.

A Yoga Secret for the Enchanting Look

One sure way to ruin your appearance every morning and for most of
the day is to eat a slowly-digesting midnight snack. No snack at all is
best, by far. Let your stomach rest from supper to breakfast, and your
face will appear far more attractive, with the least sunken cheeks, rings
under your eyes, and the aging look.

Of course, sometimes you can't help yourself and need a bedtime snack to still your appetite. Perhaps you had to skip supper. Perhaps you came home too late. Perhaps you were badly upset earlier about something or other. Perhaps you had to attend to something without delay. Perhaps you attended night school or a gym directly after work. Or countless other reasons.

For such a snack, avoid foods that require long digestion. The best of these, despite misguided popular opinion and much supposedly expert advice, is *not* stewed or cooked fruit. Eat, rather, fresh fruit without the fibrous pulp; such as grated apples or bananas. They are easy to digest. So is crushed pineapple, because it contains considerable amount of trypsin, the enzyme from your pancreas which digests meat and reduces your stomach acidity.

Avoid altogether: ham sandwiches, cocoa, milk, bread, cereals. These foods are recommended by many authorities; but the Yogis, my medical and dental ancestors and I myself, definitely *do not* recommend them for easy digestion. They stimulate the secretion of too much acid in your stomach, and make you look older next day from your body's long effort to digest them. They also fatten you easily.

Avoid cigarettes, for they have been proved to cause ulcers, probably by slowing down the neutralizing secretions from your pancreas into your stomach (probably the trypsin).

Warning: But don't eat three or four different fruits at the same snack. Being natural laxatives, they might overstimulate your bowels. Midnight snacks, in that regard, stimulate bowel action at first. But when you eat snacks regularly they contribute to constipation by depriving your stomach of the peristaltic wave stimulation which results when it is suddenly filled by a big breakfast after being empty all night. Midnight snacks, too, promote nightmares and frequent night time visits to the washroom. Crushed pineapple and a banana are perhaps the best combination snack because fresh fruits are digested rather easily. The banana "fills" you. So does the crushed pineapple due to its fiber content. It neutralizes your stomach because it contains bromelin. Bromelin is very much like trypsin or papain (from *papaya*). Best, though, *avoid snacks*.

How to Activate a Mind Recharger in Yourself

Today's labor requires less use of the bigger muscles of your body (like those of your limbs and trunk) and more use of the accessory muscle groups of your eye and hand. But these accessory muscles require large nervous output, which is increased further by the high tension you are under from the intricacy or monotony of your work. Your superior, employer, subordinate, customer, or client subconsciously detects this differing tension between your performances, and you lose out. Your blood cholesterol rises with your tension anxiety, and you are headed for hardening of the arteries. Counteract this tension anxiety with Your Mind Recharger mov-asana. Here is how to do it. (Follow Figure 27.)

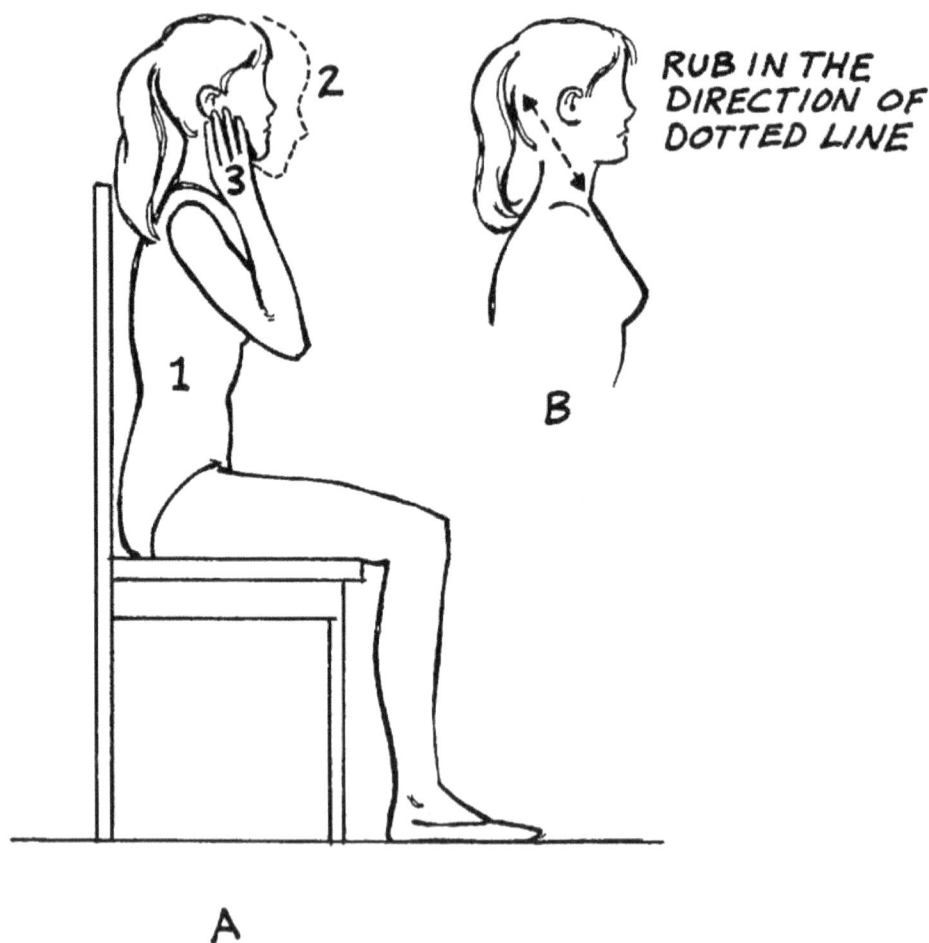

Figure 27
Your Mind Recharger

The position to assume (Figure 27A)

1. Sit straight in a chair.
2. Let your head droop forward naturally, about halfway down.

How to do this Yoga mov-asana (Figures 27A,B)

3. Place your hands against the sides of your neck, and

4. Gently rub upwards, from your neck to behind your ears (Figure 27B).

Note: Don't rub *towards* your ears. If you do, you will rub your parotid glands, and these can give you discomfort if rubbed. But by rubbing *to and behind* your ears, you easily bypass these glands. You also rub your sternomastoid muscle then and make it more pliable.

5. Turn your head to one side and rub in the same way.

6. Turn to the other side and repeat.

Frequency: Rub only twice in each position. Once a day.

What Your Mind Recharger does for you:

1. Accelerates the blood flow through your carotid arteries (which lie on the sides of your neck) *to* your brain, thereby supplying your brain with more of its main or only food—oxygen.

2. Relaxes and stretches your sternomastoid muscles (which lie on each side of your neck). That lessens their pressure against your carotid arteries and permits more blood to flow through them to your brain.

3. Your mind feels clearer fast.

4. But RUB GENTLY. Apply VERY LITTLE PRESSURE. But visualize, at the same time, the pure blood rushing faster *into* your brain, and the impure blood rushing *out* faster.

5. Your work tension-anxiety will vanish.

6. You can do this Yoga mov-asana anywhere, any time of day.

How Lorna C. Swiftly Cleared Her Frantic Mind

Lorna C. never felt at peace anymore. When she had steady work, the pressures, or the boredom or repetition, kept her either too tense or too restless. I taught Lorna Her Mind Recharger. It relaxed the muscles on each side of her neck (her sternomastoids) and let more blood reach her brain. She felt as if she had just had a good night's sleep, so fast did her mind clear. She aided the blood flow by visualizing, at the same time, the pure blood rushing faster into her brain, and the impure blood rushing out faster from it.

Happily, too, she could do the simple mov-asana any time of day, anywhere. With it she quickly cleared her mind any time it turned frantic. Her whole attitude changed. Five months later she was married to a fast-rising accountant and moved to a beautiful suburb.

How the Yoga "Enemy Crusher" Makes Your Blood Less Acid

Your conscious thinking creates baffling obstacles for you when you don't feel "good." You are filled with anger and frustration and discharge brain waves that trigger your fighting sympathetic nervous system and your adrenal glands into hyperactivity. Your blood turns more acid and you feel worse and lose out all round. Even your prospects of a promotion or a raise, are reduced. Overcome this handicap with Your Enemy Crusher mov-asana. (Follow Figure 28.)

The position to assume (Figure 28A)

1. Stand with feet one step apart, like a boxer, with

2. Left foot ahead, if you are left-handed, right foot ahead, if you are right-handed.

3. Close your fists, bend your elbows, and draw your arms against your sides, like a boxer.

How to do this Yoga mov-asana (Figures 28 B,C,D)

4. Visualize your "bad" conscious thinking standing before you like someone you don't know. Recall how frequently it holds you back in your work or daily activity.

5. Poke at it with your left fist (or right fist if you are left-handed) as if to hold it off at striking distance.

6. Step 4 inches forwards with your left foot (your front foot, Figure 28C) and

7. Slap the image of your "bad" conscious thinking viciously with your right hand. Swing at it with your right fist if you prefer, but don't strike the furniture. "Hit," nonetheless, to get the rage out of your system.

8. Visualize the image of your "bad" conscious thinking crumble from the blow.

9. "See" it get up again and attack you (Figure 28D).

10. But poke and slap (or hit) it again, and floor it again.

11. Repeat the whole procedure 3 times.

Frequency: 3 repetitions. 1 set (group of repetitions). Every working day.

What Your Enemy Crusher does for you:

1. You feel like a different person altogether.

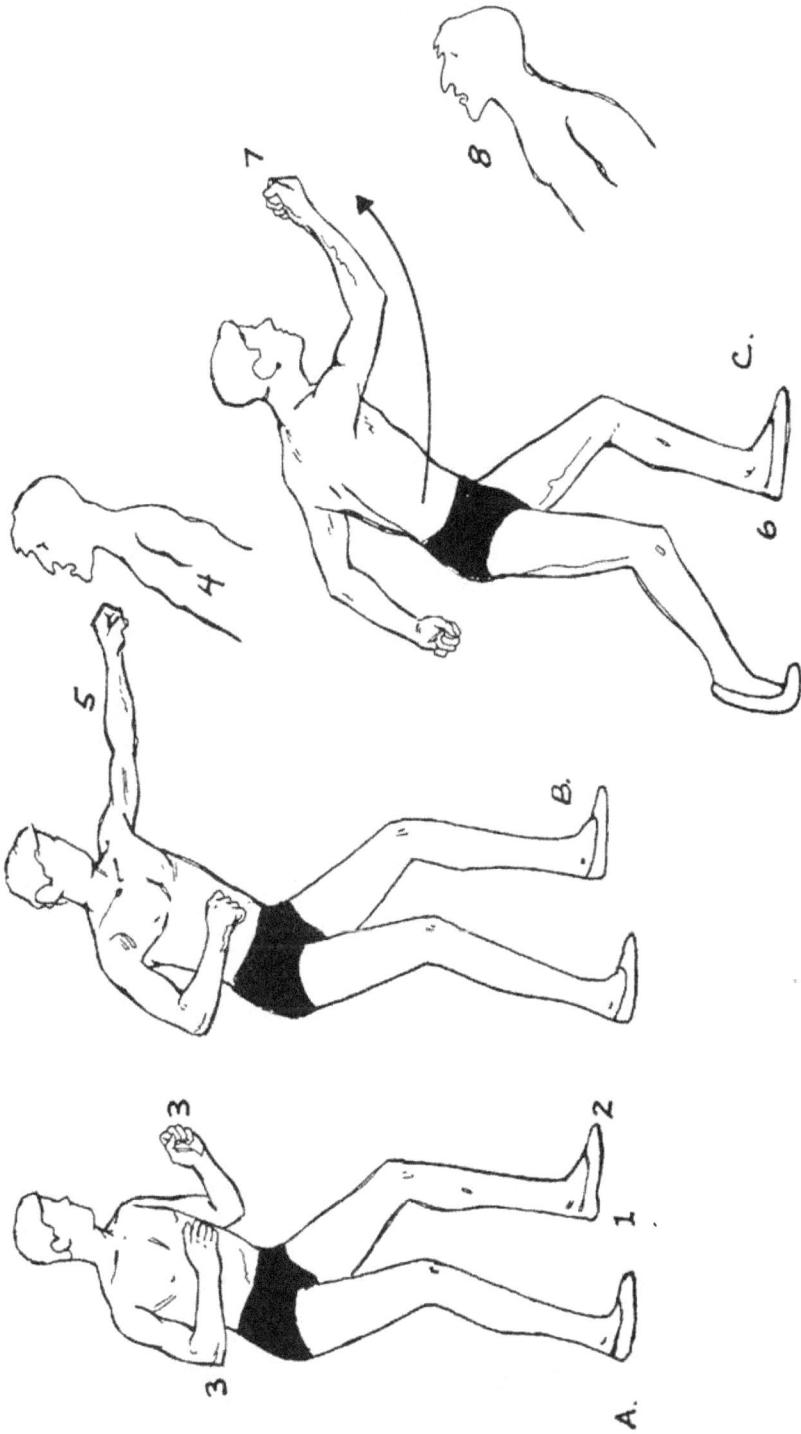

Figure 28
Your Enemy Crusher

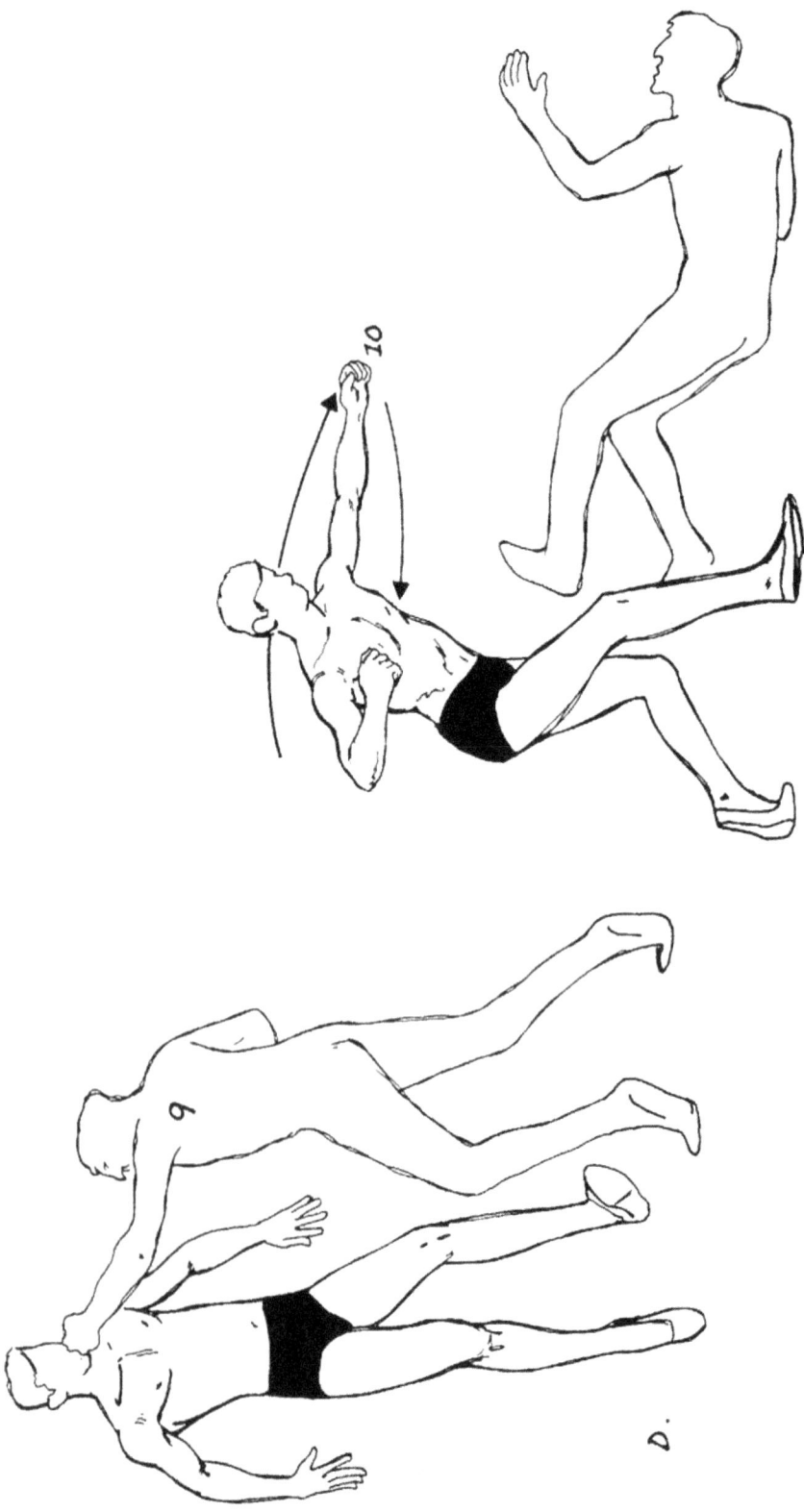

Figure 28, cont.

2. Your anger and frustration depart, and your conscious mind discharges brain waves which trigger your *para*sympathetic nervous system and your thyroid glands. Your blood turns less acidic soon afterwards.

3. Your prospects of promotion, or of a raise, are considerably increased.

How to use Your Enemy Crusher mov-asana in your everyday life:

1. Aware yourself of this brain wave of yours sometime after doing this Yoga mov-asana. Reproduce it by feeling *exactly as you felt* after knocking down the image of your "bad" conscious thinking (in the mirror) the second time.

2. After a little practice you will reproduce this brain wave of yours at will *any time at work* or in any other activity.

3. You will succeed in it as you never have before, even when you don't feel "good."

How Jack H. Overthrew His Desperation

Business competition was getting Jack H. down. It was his habit to do his best in everything, but the company he worked for had been losing money steadily. Jack felt cornered, with enemies on every side ready to make a scapegoat of him and oust him. The stigma that he had "failed the company" would undermine his chances of landing another good position. For the last three years his mind was in a turmoil. He could hardly think straight anymore, he said.

At his insistence I taught Jack His Enemy Crusher mov-asana. After battering to the ground, in his very first workout, the images of his "bad" conscious thinking about his "enemies," Jack felt like a different person. His anger and frustration vanished, and his conscious mind discharged brain waves which triggered his peace-loving *para*sympathetic nervous system and his thyroid glands. Jack reproduced that brain wave sometime later by feeling *exactly as he felt* after knocking down the images of his "bad" conscious thinking.

At the company he reproduced that same brain wave at will, *anytime* he needed it. To his relief, the pressures against him relaxed. Support for his policies increased, and the Board agreed to back his revolutionary plans for a company comeback. The plans worked rather effectively, and Jack got a nice promotion and a thrilling raise.

Reducing Your Anxieties with Graceful Movement

Running away from your anxieties may be the best treatment possible (Morgan).[1] Scientists had warned people, for a long time, not to exercise to try to relieve their anxieties. Exercise, they explained, would intensify their anxieties because it increased their blood lactate level, a factor in their bodies which increased during anxiety. For 40 years I myself preached and taught *the very opposite view*. Scientists are now agreeing all-out with me.[2] *Now* they are believing that exercise *reduces* anxiety.

My research, both on myself and on many people for nearly 45 years, has proved to me that exercise, *if not done excessively for too long workouts*, REDUCES anxiety. The powerful muscle contractions which you make in violent exercise rid your body fastest of anxiety for about 24 hours. That's why the person with a speech impediment, like stuttering and stammering, speaks most fluently *for hours* after engaging in violent exercise which does not exhaust him. (If it exhausts him, he speaks worse until next day).

The same principle applies to you. Run away from your anxiety by sprinting at top speed for a short distance. Stop before exhausting yourself and walk about two to three times the same distance before sprinting again. After four or five such sprints and walks, return home and do your favorite Yoga mov-asanas. *Do only your favorite ones*, so as to feel thoroughly liberated. The moment you feel bored (as everyone eventually does with anything he repeats constantly), exercise no more that day. Rest on your back, then, for a half hour. *That's* how to relieve your anxieties with your muscles.

Note: If it is inconvenient (and sometimes even unsafe) for you to go outdoors and sprint do The Torso Push (page 36-38). Resist hard the push of your legs and do about 5-6 repetitions. Or resist the push only hard enough to let you do about 20 repetitions. (This mov-asana exercises your thighs like running.) Then stretch your back with Your Sacro-Stretch (page 201) to lengthen it and relieve compressions of your spinal nerves, and feel "light" again.

How the Housewife Syndrome Converts You into a Pitiful Wreck

Housework tends to isolate you from the world, for you do it in small, private living units. If you have young children, up to as old as teenagers, they restrict your freedom severely. Housework, besides, is repetitious and subjects you abnormally to dust, noise (vacuum cleaner, laundry machine, etc.), noxious fumes (from polishing fluids, detergents, and other chemicals), physical strains and uncomfortable positions, periods of long standing, and of fatigue and other unhealthy side effects. From the labor standpoint it is basically menial work, no matter what you call it. Much of it, besides, leads to chronic ill-health. Too much of it requires you to bend and twist at the waist after your meals, paving the road for chronic indigestion and migraine headaches. Eventually, the repetitious movements and unavoidable strains can afflict you with bursitis of one or both shoulders, arthritis of your back (particularly, of your lower back), so-called sciatic neuritis, and painless pathologies like varicose veins.

Housework is labor, not systematic exercise. Systematic exercise beautifies your body by altering its contours for the better. That's one important reason for doing the Yoga mov-asanas. Housework, in contrast, robs you of youth and beauty. It does little for your waist (except to let it sag and spread bigger), or for your shoulders (except to overwork them and let them droop). Just because you are weary at the end of a long housekeeping chore does not mean that you have exercised systematically with benefit to your health and figure.

Unlike proper exercise, also, housework, according to researchers, encourages you to brood, leading you to form erratic judgments about many of your problems and to acquire mental aberrations and a sense of powerlessness. You try to complete the boresome task as soon as possible and have time left for something more pleasant and inspiring. Housework diminishes your sexual attractions, and leads you into the housewife's syndrome. In this syndrome you feel nervous and have difficulty falling asleep. Your hands tremble and perspire. You suffer from nightmares; you feel faint, headachy and dizzy, and shake from heart palpitations. You become dissatisfied with life. You pine for a job outside the home so you could go out daily, dressed up stylishly, instead of hustling between the same four walls from sunup to sundown and away from the excitement of the world, getting "old" and fat and being forgotten by the rest of humanity. Learn how to overcome this dreaded syndrome and gain in beauty and health from being a housewife.

How to Overcome the Housewife Syndrome and Gain in Health and Beauty

It is not unnatural to be a housewife. So, stop worrying about it if you are one. Worrying can sicken you. Stop complaining about how "filthy" everybody else in the house is. Stop worrying, when you fall prey to it, about the family's unpaid bills, the long-lasting home mortgage, your children's disappointing grades, your husband's "not-big-enough" pay. Stop pining for the numerous household "gadgets" you wish you had but "can't afford" to get; the fancy vacation you might have to cancel for lack of enough cash, and so on, and so on.

Pause and rest every hour or so during your housekeeping day by sitting or lying down for ten minutes. (But don't lie down for two hours after a heavy meal, or for one and one-half hours after a light one.) Change periodically, too, from standing housework to sitting housework and rest your legs, your back, your shoulders and your dragged down rib-box from the merciless downpull of gravity. And before resuming the chore, do three or four repetitions of Your Sacro-Stretch (page 201) to relieve your spinal nerves from the excessive squeeze down on them by your vertebrae, also due to the merciless downpull of gravity. Even lie down, if you are empty enough, and do The Myotatic Relaxer, (page 27).

The next time you rest sitting down, do Your Rude Awakener (page 203) to tone up your back muscles and relieve your shoulders from the wearisome contest against gravity. Before you stand up again, too, massage your calves a little, rubbing them from the ankles upwards to help the blood return to your heart. Kneed gently the bulkiest portions of your calf muscles to encourage still more the stagnating circulation in the veins of your calves to move upwards towards your heart, instead of pressing back down into your ankles and, in time, swelling them.

Even elevate your legs for a few minutes while lying down and resting, upon two pillows piled on top each other, and with a rolled blanket under your knees to keep them slightly bent.

To rest on your back while lying down, let your heels hang loose beyond the edge of the mattress. And, again, place a rolled blanket or a pillow under your knees to keep them slightly bent. It will prevent them from straining their joints or tightening and tensing the muscles at the backs of your thighs.

On days when you do less housework, do more Yoga mov-asanas to restore the vanishing beauty of your body and prevent it from degenerating into that of a housewife-matron. The movements and stimulations of these Yoga secrets will thrill you, and the housewife syndrome will lose its grip on you. You will gain more then than you lose physically and mentally from the chores of housekeeping.

Developing a Jupiter Lift to Raise Your Mood

How you start off your day has a decisive bearing upon how you make out the rest of the day. If you start off not feeling at your most capable, most cheerful, most energetic, most determined, most glamorous, or most rested, you will most likely live through a wretched day of missed opportunities, friends lost, romance thwarted, work badly done, or even be involved in accidents. The Yogis were masters at starting their *seven days a week* right. They had so many plans to perfect the different powers of their minds and bodies that they had little time to waste. The Jupiter Lift is the simple, non-tiring, effective scientific Yoga mov-asana to throw you into your best mood at the beginning of the day. It is the mov-asana (moving posture) to make every day of your life a perfect one in every way. Here is how to do it. (Follow Figure 29.)

The Jupiter Lift

The position to assume (Figure 29A)

1. Stand with feet about 10-14 inches apart, knees slightly bent, and back slightly crouched, as if you are ready to jump.
2. Hold arms out at sides, elbows bent,
3. Palms down, but relaxed.

How to do this Yoga mov-asana

4. Swing your bent arms around *in a circle*. Swing them around first backwards and upwards (when they will tense). Then continue swinging them forwards and downwards (when they will relax) (Figures 29 A,B,C).

Note: Actually your *shoulders* swing. Your arms go along with them.

5. Inhale as you swing "them" backwards and upwards (Figure 29B).
6. Exhale as you swing them forwards and downwards (Figure 29C).
7. Swing them fast and vigorously—but completely! Make *full circles* with your shoulders.
8. Bend your knees up and down naturally with the swings.

Frequency: 7 repetitions. 2 sets (groups of repetitions). 3 times a week. Swing and rotate your shoulders around, like a bird about to "take off" and fly.

What the Jupiter Lift does for you (Figure 29D)

1. Proportions your shoulders and shapes your upper back where you are likely to acquire a middle-age padding of excess flesh (especially if you are a woman).
2. Throws you into the best mood at the very beginning of the day to combine "boring" detail with bubbling enthusiasm. You will draw to you one

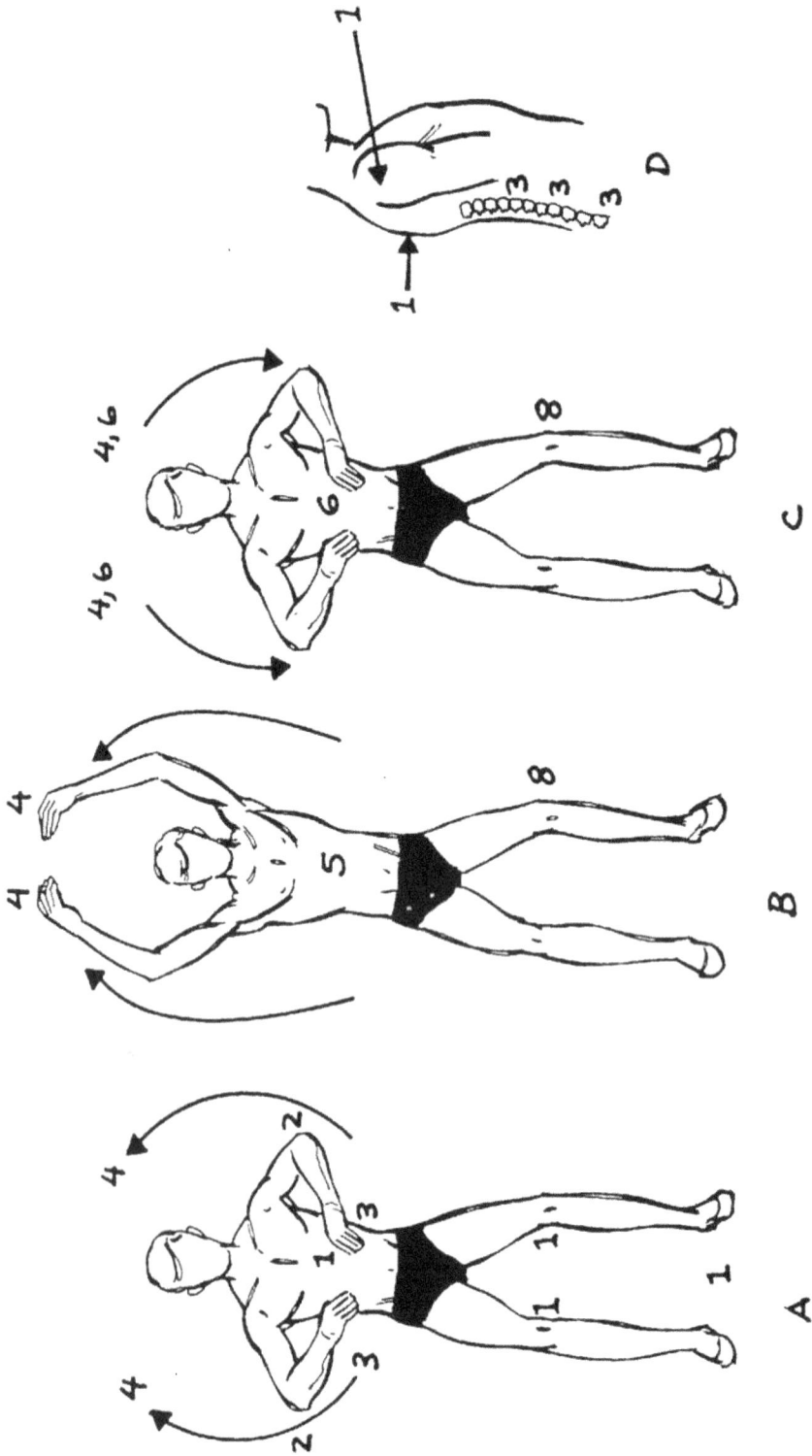

Figure 29
The Jupiter Lift

lucky break after another.

3. Stimulates the vertebrae of your lower back (1-4 lumbar) and your sacrum and coccyx. That improves your uterus, bladder, legs.

How Betty N. Felt "Like a Million Bucks"

Betty N. was diagnosed as being healthy enough for a normal person. But she had difficulty getting up in the mornings. And after she did, she felt lackadaisical, uninspired, and ready to go back to bed, as if she had slept all night in an airless closet. She left home grouchy and made enemies at every turn. People who saw her or dealt with her thought that she was much older than she was. She was even acquiring a middle-age padding of excess flesh on her shoulders and upper back, and it made her even more sullen.

I taught Betty The Jupiter Lift. The rotary arm movement and her whole body participation filled her with eagerness and excitement. In a little over a week the mov-asana was noticeably proportioning her shoulders and shaping her upper arms. It was also shaving the "fat hump" off her upper back. She felt the thrill all down her body, in fact, for the "gaiety" of the movement stimulated her lower back and legs, too. Betty felt like an athlete or a dancer ready to put on a masterpiece performance.

She thrilled everybody, now, on her way to work and *at* work. And people remarked that she looked amazingly younger.

Yoga Meditation Exercises for Superior Mental Concentration

Daily, you face delicate situations with people in your career and in your home which cannot be ironed out with sheer logic or factual evidence. Such situations require the use of a sixth sense. But your emotions and prejudiced logic paralyze your instinctive attempts to do whatever is necessary. They are under the influence of your out-of-beat physiological rhythms, which depend upon the biological time of day. Your out-of-beat rhythms shatter your power of superior mental concentration.

Counteract those evils with the Yoga meditation mov-asana. Acquire with it a sixth sense, or a power of superior mental concentration, which synchronizes the right circadian rhythms in you at *any time* of the day, regardless of your biological clock. It will bury your prejudiced logic and your emotions and open up to you vistas of thinking to which you were previously blind. With such a staggering power of meditation you will astonish others—*and yourself*—by seeing the practically *un*perceivable in anything you undertake. The secret mov-asana for this is The Crack Skull. (Follow Figure 30).

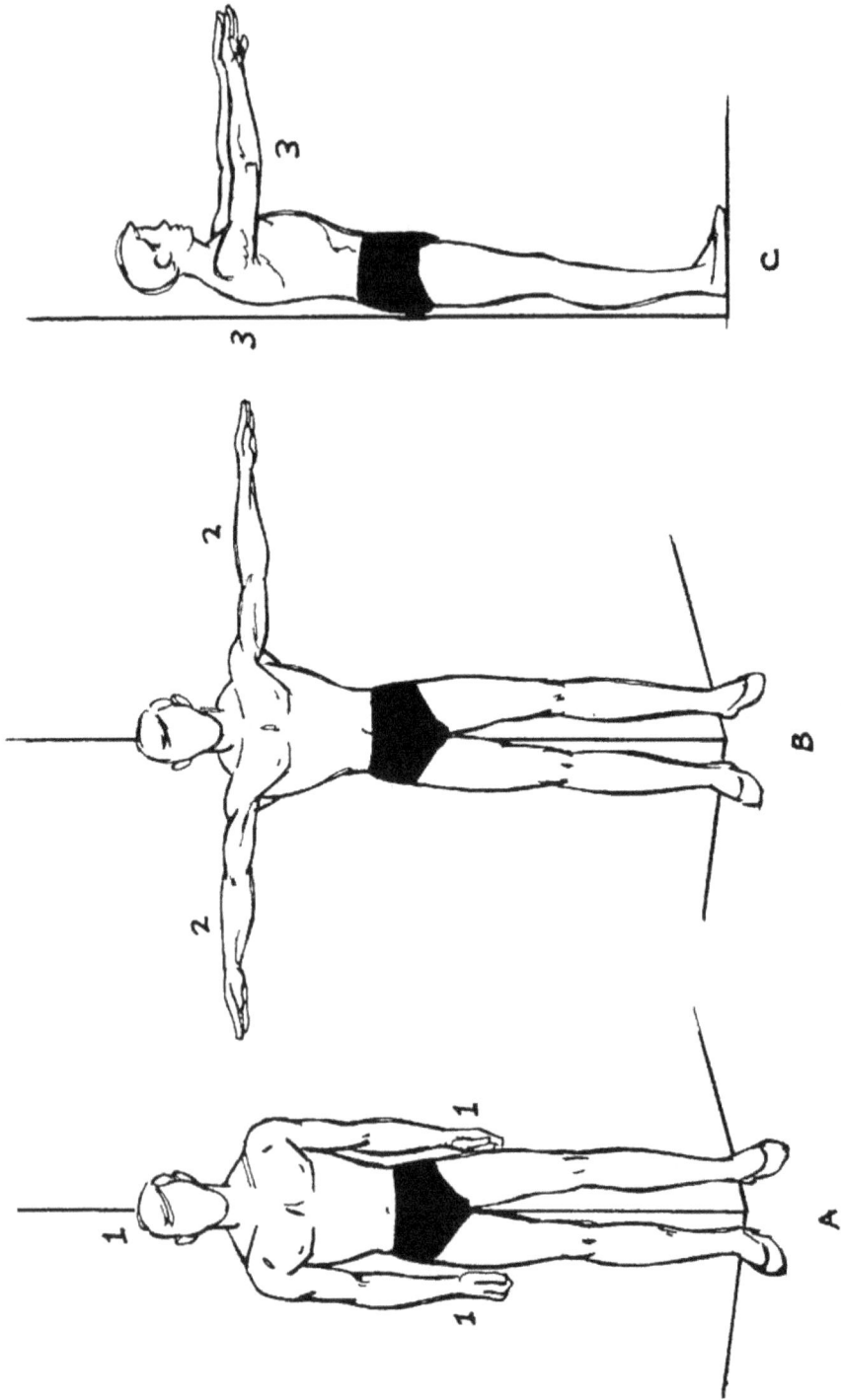

Figure 30
The Crack Skull

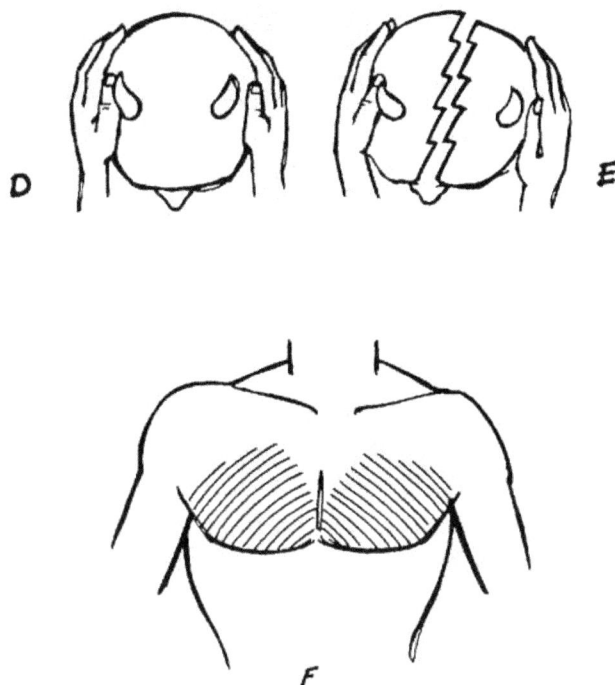

Figure 30, cont.

The Power of the Crack Skull

The position to assume (Figure 30A)

1. Stand against a corner of a doorway in your home, with arms hanging by your sides.

How to do this Yoga mov-asama (Figure 30B)

2. Fill yourself with fear of something you dread greatly. Open your arms at shoulder level to suggest helplessness to your mind. Opening your arms uses your muscles of surrender. The corner of the doorway pressing against your back helps to keep you balanced. You feel like a dependent person when you open your arms. Now,

3. Round your back (Figure 30C). Partly bend your arms and bring them partly forwards together. Visualize them squeezing a giant Satanic skull, until they crush it down to human size by the time they extend to arm's length (Figure 30D).

4. Tense your chest muscles (or breasts) tightly as you do so (Figure 30F).

5. Compress that now life-sized skull fiercely—and crack it (Figure 30E).

Frequency: 4 repetitions. 1 set (group of repetitions). 4 times a week.

What The Crack Skull does for you (Figure 30F)

1. Fills and firms the whole of your chest muscles (or breasts).

2. Cracking the imaginary skull jars your out-of-beat physiological (circadian) rhythms *into synchrony with each other*.

3. It thereby stabilizes your biological clock considerably all day and brings you a staggering power to meditate and solve the most baffling problems.

How Curt F. Broke Away from His Volcanic Upsets Forever

Curt F. was desperate. No matter how thoroughly he prepared to meet any important situation, when he faced it he seemed to fly apart and fail miserably. He was diagnosed as normal, but I suspected that his circadian rhythms synchronized only when he was at peace. The moment he faced others for something important, his different circadian rhythms went off their own ways and left him a floundering hulk.

I taught Curt The Crack Skull. In the imagined skull he visualized his volcanic emotions impeding his every move in life. He compressed the skull fiercely—and "cracked" it. The moment he did so he felt a big change within him, as if his different body parts now suddenly fit together and functioned in concert. His out-of-beat circadian rhythms, in other words, had been jarred into synchrony with each other.

At the end of the set, Curt felt that there was nothing in the world he could not do. His hands throbbed with the feeling of victory, and reflexly the sensation flashed to his brain. His superior at work detected the new man in him. Six months later Curt landed the highest post in his department.

Achieving Confidence and Serenity That Can Add Years to Your Life

Your modern environment strains your nerves and your big skeletal muscles. As a result, your natural alertness gives way to irritability, leaving you emotional. When you are under the influence of emotion, powerful chemical substances pour from your organs into your tissues and can rob you of confidence and serenity, and shorten your life.[3] Psychiatrists have even induced attacks of the painful state of fear by injecting patients with lactic acid, a chemical substance which is increased in your bloodstream after exercise.

That is why your reactions to stress are so strongly influenced by your diet. When you adopt a low-fat, *low* cholesterol diet, sad to admit, you *reduce* your body's ability to handle stress. With foods *high* in cholesterol, in contrast, animals (and humans) perform *better* under stress than on a low-fat diet. A diet containing *fatty foods*, like cream, bacon, or grated raw cocoanut, add a warm padding of fat throughout your body and tranquilize you. A *low*-fat diet, however, deprives you of this warm padding of fat and puts you physically "in the pink," but leaves you mentally on edge and hyper-reactive under stress. That is why a *fat-rich* diet, although it heightens your possibilities of suffering a heart attack earlier, *also increases your capacity to handle stress*. It explains why you feel so much calmer after eating pecans or raw cocoanut with your meals for several days. But you will have also increased your blood cholesterol level.

If your blood pressure is normal enough, then, and if you are still not above middle-age, you may have to resort to such a diet periodically for a few days when you are burdened with stress in order to meet tense situations more calmly. But you should return to a more normal diet afterwards without delay! It is wise, though, to resort to the secret Yoga mov-asana to acquire confidence and serenity swiftly. This mov-asana is The Lactic Releaser. Here is how to do it. (No accompanying illustration.)

1. Sit before your mirror and accept your reflected image as being that of the person you wish to impress. It may be your superior at work, your subordinate, your loved one, your offspring, or some stranger.

2. Due to the excessive emotional reactions you have acquired towards your modern environment, you dread not being able to influence that person as you wish. As a result you do fail to influence him (or her).

3. Your fear-sympathetics (the "fear portion" of your sympathetic nervous system) speed up your heart and turn your breathing fast and shallow. At the same time, glycogen in your liver is converted to sugar to supply more energy to your now poised-for-action muscles. These muscles use up this sugar and cast off lactic acid as a waste product. Since injections of lactic acid induce anxiety in animals, this added lactic acid in your bloodstream *increases* your excessive emotions.

4. *Prevent* your emotions from increasing by *lessening* the amount of this added lactic acid accumulating in your bloodstream. To achieve that:

5. Take a half breath, and hold it for four seconds.

6. By then you will be gasping for breath. It will stimulate your fear-sympathetics still more by frightening you with the prospects of suffocation.

7. Then exhale quietly and breathe normally again.

8. Your subconscious mind will respond now as if you have *already* faced the person or obstacle in the mirror and overcome him or it. The added lactic acid

in you will be thrown off through your lungs in the form of carbon dioxide. Your fear-sympathetics, as a result, will lose their abnormal drive to protect you. And so, your irritability will be reduced markedly.

Frequency: Do this secret Yoga mov-asana 5 times every morning. Do it easily any time during the day. It also helps to stabilize your heart and normalize your blood pressure.

How Lou E. Suddenly Swept Others off Their Feet

No matter how thoroughly Lou E. prepared himself to impress others, the moment he faced them, his heart pounded so hard that he could hardly breathe. His forehead blazed with heat, and his body turned rigid. He became a veritable nobody. He envied calm people who swept others off their feet.

I taught Lou the Lactic Releaser. After practicing it *only once* he was a changed person. Next day he faced the very person he wanted to impress most with a new, calm repose, for his subconscious mind responded as if he had *already* swept that person off his feet. Lou's emotionality was ousted, and he carried his plans through with thrilling exactitude.

References

[1]Professor William Morgan of the University of Wisconsin. *Science Digest*, July, 1973.

[2]Dr. Herbert De Vries, physiologist at the University of Southern California. At a meeting of the American College of Sports Medicine.

[3]Dr. George Engel, psychologist at the University of Rochester, New York.

Dr. Martin Seligman, psychologist at the University of Pennsylvania.

9

How Yoga Gives You
A Youthfully, Healthful Digestive System

The Yoga "Toning up" Effect on Stomach and Intestines

As exercise, the Yoga mov-asanas have an added advantage over lifting weights because you can perform them from positions which would be unsafe or impossible with weights. To handle barbells you have to sit, stand, or lie in positions which permit the weight to be supported or suspended mainly by your skeleton. The weight you could manage safely, otherwise, would be too light to bring benefits. With the Yoga mov-asanas, though, you can vary the resistance you have to overcome in the movement with your own counter muscles, with the balls of your feet, with your knees, with your skeletal leverage, with changing the angles of using your joints, and other natural mechanisms. And you can do so from so many different angles that you can alter the contours of any part of your body with comparative ease.

The same applies to your stomach and intestines. The Yoga mov-asanas brace your abdominal muscles and massage your stomach from easy positions without the painful contractions resulting from using barbells or apparatus, thus adding pleasure to the exertion. This pleasure stimulates your stomach and intestines and tones them up, so that you look forward to them with excitement rather than with dread. Your parasympathetic nervous system—the nervous system of your normal functions—is triggered by pleasure and rushes more nerve-electricity to your stomach and intestines and gives them more tone.

The Yoga mov-asanas, besides, arouse your sympathetic nervous system less than barbells or apparatus because they spare you from the feeling of performing something heavily laborious, so your stomach and intestines remain toned up more than normally. That's the Yoga secret.

161

Effect of the Splanchnic Double-Curl After You Eat

Over the years your sympathetic nervous system experiences many shocks. You grow distrustful of other people because you see shrewd dishonesty of so many of the people on the job, in business, or socially, or romantically. Your outraged sympathetic nervous system turns you secretly hostile and plagues you with digestion tension. Many other conditions likewise affect your system, such as unhappiness, disappointment, financial worry, losing your job, the unexplainable desertion of friends, the breaking of your engagement to marry, the discovery that your mate is unfaithful, a divorce, the death of a loved one. Even subclinical pains in your middle back flash their undiagnosable irritations continuously to your conscious mind and turn you into a more easily-provoked, hastily-acting person, particularly when confronted with an exasperating situation.

The resulting digestion tension "nails" you to the "vagaries" of your stomach. It also overtones the muscles attached to your 5-6-7-8 dorsal vertebrae (or the vertebrae in the middle portion of your back) and ruins the flexibility of those vertebral joints.

Use the secret Yoga mov-asana The Splanchnic Double-Curl to relieve this digestion tension in you—and restore the lost acuity of your mind. Here is how to do it. (Follow Figure 31.)

The position to assume (Figure 31A)

1. Stand straight, with heels about 1½ feet apart, and toes pointing normally slightly outwards.

2. Raise your arms above your head and clasp your hands together.

How to do the First Curl of this Yoga mov-asana (Figure 31B)

3. Swing your arms (with hands still clasped) far down to between your knees.

4. Bend your knees as you do so, and

5. Draw in your waist tight.

How to do the Second Curl of this Yoga mov-asana (Figure 31C)

6. Unclasp your hands and fold your arms behind your head, as in Number 8, but do it bent over, in position for Number 6. Now,

7. Raise your body to a straight-up position. Your middle (and lower) back muscles tighten to lift your torso back to the erect. That is the Second Curl. Now,

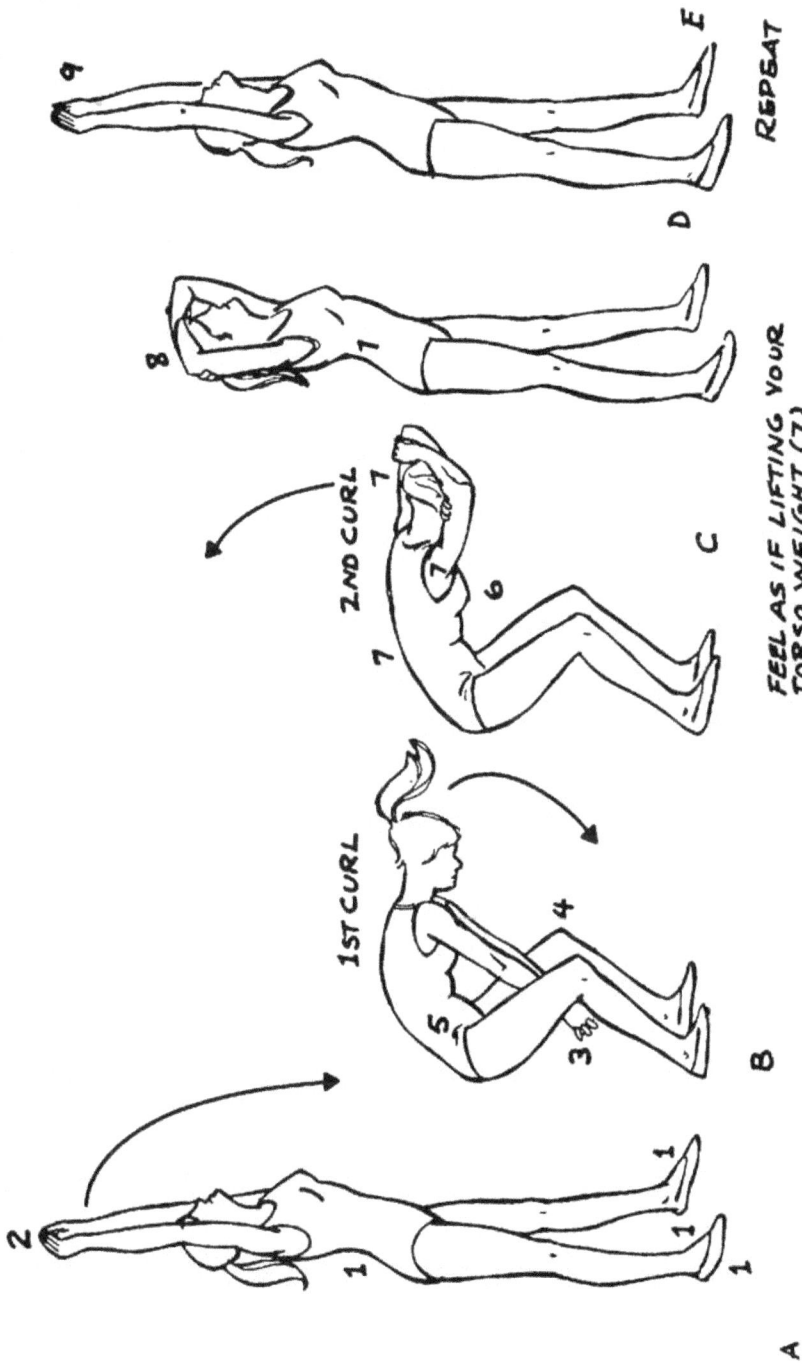

FEEL AS IF LIFTING YOUR
TORSO WEIGHT (7)
Figure 31
The Splanchic Double-Curl

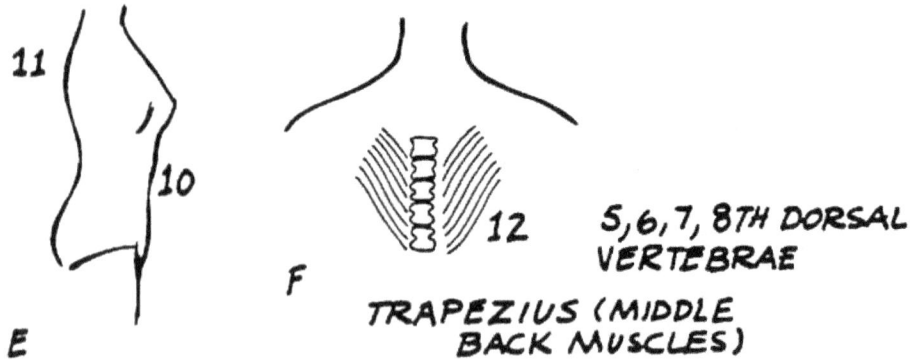

11

10

12   **5,6,7, 8TH DORSAL VERTEBRAE**

F

TRAPEZIUS (MIDDLE BACK MUSCLES)

E

Figure 31, cont.

8. Straighten your arms overhead, clasp your hands together again, and repeat the whole movement, starting from A.

What The Splanchnic Double-Curl does for you (Figure 31E,F)

    1. Draws in and flattens your waistline.

    2. Balances the contours of your middle back.

    3. Stimulates the nerves passing between your 5,6,7,8 dorsal vertebrae and thereby improves your liver, pancreas, stomach and small intestines.

How Linda H. Ended Her After-Meal Upsets

Linda H. had developed an "allergy" to the dinner table. No matter how hungry she felt, the prospect of eating a meal threw her into near panic. Her food didn't "settle well" in her. Instead of feeling better after eating, she felt bloated, sluggish, belched easily, and was heavy in the right side, even headachy. Thorough clinical tests found nothing organically wrong with her, except that her digestion was very sensitive.

I taught Linda The Splanchnic Double-Curl. Although she noted little change at first, in a month she enjoyed her meals more and more, and her digestion was less sensitive. She was losing her dread of the dinner table and the consequent discomfort that followed it. Her waistline, meanwhile, was being drawn in and flattened. Her middle back, too, was acquiring beautiful contours.

A few weeks later Linda confessed that at last she was enjoying eating without after-meal upsets. She called it a miracle.

Caution: Do no abdominal mov-asana less than 2¼ hours after a light meal (fruit and salad), or less than 3 hours after a heavy meal.

Secrets to Avoid Kidney Infection

Next to your brain and your heart, your kidneys are the most impor-tant organs you have. When they start malfunctioning you feel tired, your blood pressure rises, your appetite departs, your sleep lessens, your legs twitch, your skin bruises more easily, and headaches come. You feel listless, and might even vomit in the morning. Taking large doses of vitamin C for colds, besides masking early signs of liver trouble, can curse you with kidney stones. Even a strep throat, if not cleared up quickly, causes your body to release antibodies to attack the germs, and these can also attack your kidneys and cause them to break down. Even cavities in your teeth can cause your kidneys to break down, for when you "chew" on the cavities, you can push bacteria through them into your bloodstream and bring on kidney inflammation.

Your customary daily diet may be injurious, leading to inflammation of your intestines (enteritis) and thus contribute to kidney infection. This, in turn, could produce more irritation to your kidneys from the toxic substances and bacteria which are absorbed in increased amounts from your disordered intestines. Insufficient daily intake of plain water adds further to your misery by permitting the constant presence of certain salts in your urine, like oxalates, which might even cause kidney stones. The foods you eat, usually containing sugar, could even bring on a state in you similar to the sugar in the blood in diabetes and irritate your kidneys still further. Even if you are so little sickened in this manner that your condi-tion eludes diagnosis, you still suffer from loss of vitality.

It is wise, then, to eat balanced meals with plenty of fruits and vegetables. Erroneously-called "acid" fruits, like pineapples, oranges and grapefruits, as stated previously, actually *alkalize* your stomach to an alkaline state. Eat no more than six ounces of meat a day. Avoid all tea, coffee, liquors, and artificial stimulants. But drink from six to eight glasses of plain water a day, *in addition* to your meal-time liquids. Avoid fatty foods, like bacon, cocoanuts, Brazil nuts, ham, too much pork.

Fluids a Yogi Uses for Kidney Stones

I taught this program to my followers and published it early in the

1950's. Twenty years later, in 1974, Dr. Ruben Gittes, professor and head of the Urology Division of the University of California at San Diego, revealed at the American College of Surgeons Clinical Congress that people prone to kidney stones should drink at least eight glasses of water—or drinks containing water—every day. Dr. Birdwell Finlayson, professor of urological surgery at the University of Florida, agreed with him. Dr. Gittes called nonsense the "very rigid diet on which some doctors" put their patients, telling them not to eat a long li of foods, ranging from pancakes, certain fruits, seafood, pea soup, molasses, and many vegetables. "Drinking water is the really important thing," he declared. His views differed from mine, though, by accepting soft drinks, tea, or even beer in place of water.

He advises against consuming dairy products containing lactose, such as milk and cheese, because lactose promotes calcium absorption, and both doctors agree that too much calcium in the blood causes kidney stones. My own researches do not support milk as a cause of kidney stone. But I advise you, if you have "bad" kidneys, not to eat too much food containing oxalic or phytic acid. Such foods, in excess, could cause kidney stones. Among these are prunes, tomatoes, rhubarb, spinach, cereals, and beans. A Mexican scientist even added beets and celery to the list. Foods that contain the most calcium, ironically, also contain oxalic or phytic acid. Orange and grapefruit and grapefruit juice are known, by the Yogis, to dissolve kidney stone.

Note: But see your doctor or healer first, of course, because in certain types of "bad" kidneys, the water cannot filter through the kidney. You would have to *abstain* from liquids then.

The Secret Yogi Practice, Made Scientific, to Discourage an Acid Stomach

To discourage an acid stomach is not easy. But the Yogis were excellent at doing so, particularly with their power of mind-over-matter. The American Medical Association upholds them with its discoveries that people with peptic ulcers are helped almost as much by placebos (sugar-coated, non-medical pills) as by popular calcium carbonate antacids.

But the Yogis don't always combat stomach upsets with their minds alone. They add a ritual to the process. My medical ancestors refined this ritual into a science and used it successfully in their practice.

This is the Yogi secret, made scientific. When you suffer from stomach trouble:

1. Eat nothing for a whole day.

2. Take two enemas that day. Take one upon arising, and the other late in

the afternoon. Lie on your back when taking them, with your knees bent close up to your chest. Massage your abdomen thoroughly to percolate the enema water as high as possible into your three colons. Retain each of the two enemas as long as possible before letting them out.

3. Drink, that day, two or three glasses of water every hour.

4. Rest for hours lying on your left side, with a moist heating pad against your abdomen. It relaxes your acid-contracted abdominal muscles and your pyloric valve (the valve which shuts off the farther end of your stomach and keeps the undigested food in it). The water you drank will drain out of your stomach through your pyloric valve and carry your excessive gastric acids into your small intestines and leave your stomach neutralized.

5. As you rest on your left side, visualize all these scenes occurring. Visualize the farther end of your stomach (your pyloric valve) opening, and the water you drank washing all the acid in your stomach out of it. Visualize this water streaming through your intestines and colon. . . flooding your rectum. . . being evacuated from it and leaving your stomach and your alimentary canal clean and no longer acidic. Visualize all this so clearly that you get the "feeling" in your brain. The "feeling" will release its own brain waves all through you and encourage still more complete evacuation. You will be adding the power of mind-over-matter to your evacuation, and the enema will prove to be far more effective, as the American Medical Association found to be the case with placebos.

6. By next day you will feel "miraculously" better.

A Yoga Visceral Controller That Soothes an Acid Stomach Quickly

Your digestive system is strongly under the control of your emotions. "Heartburn" is brought on by hyperacidity of your stomach, and among its causes are excitement, emotion, certain foods, drinking certain liquors, or smoking certain brands of tobacco. Whatever the cause of your "bad" stomach, it triggers your sympathetic nervous system into action. Your brain, as a result, throws out brain waves of anxiety which stimulate your fear-sympathetics to slow down your digestion. When, like the Yogis, you control your emotions, you are closer to insuring yourself a healthy stomach. The Yoga mov-asana to achieve that is Your Visceral Brain Wave Controller. Here is how to do it. (No figure is necessary).

The position to assume

1. Take a sheet of newspaper which would require, say, ten minutes to read. But

2. Allow yourself only seven or eight minutes to read it.

3. You doubt whether you can read it in time, so you determine to rush through it.

4. This decision fills you with tension. Your sympathetic nervous system is triggered and your digestion slowed.

5. Your brain responds by creating the brain waves of tension.

How to do this Yoga mov-asana.

6. Hold the sheet of newspaper before you again and assure yourself that you WILL read it in time. Tell yourself that you *will* peruse it at a normal pace, but that you will waste no time while doing it.

7. And yet, should you *fail to* read it in time, you *won't care!*

8. Start to read the newspaper with this attitude. Don't race against time, just read normally. Try to understand all you read that you consider important. But pass by the seemingly unimportant details. Watch the clock, but don't grow alarmed if your pace lags behind it.

9. *Don't skim* over insignificant facts, though. Nothing tenses you more than skimming over what you wish to understand clearly, but hurriedly. It routs your brain waves of calm.

10. After reading in that manner for about five minutes, your brain will be discharging your natural brain wave of concentrating without tension.

11. Under the influence of your *natural brain wave*, the secretion of your gastric (digestive) juices returns to normal.

12. This natural brain wave is *your* visceral brain wave controller. It is the brain wave which controls all your visceral organs and keeps them healthy, providing that you don't abuse them with improper eating and living habits.

13. Fifteen minutes later try to feel *exactly* as you felt when doing number 12, or with your *natural brain wave*. Practice getting that feeling several times during the day, so that you can feel that way *at will*.

14. To retain normal digestion, feel like that every time you eat, and after you eat. You will create Your Visceral Brain Wave Controller, and your stomach will remain healthy year after year.

How Andrew B. Conquered His Stomach Upsets

Andrew B. belched noticeably after eating, and suffered, even while still eating, from crawling headaches. They commenced at the left side of his head and climbed upward, along where he parted his hair. He also experienced annoying, creeping sensations around his temples. They were unpleasant and bewildered him. His doctor told him that he had a very sensitive stomach, either innately or acquired through his diet or his life habits.

I taught Andrew His Visceral Brain Wave Controller. He could have acquired his sensitive stomach, as I had long ago discovered, from habitually overconcentrating with his mind on "everything" he did.

His Visceral Brain Wave Controller mov-asana was so different from what Andrew had expected of Yoga that he didn't believe me at first. He tried it, nonetheless. After doing it for five minutes, though, he was already aware that he was mentally concentrating *without* tension. His brain, in other words, was discharging *his natural* brain wave, and the secretions of his gastric (digestive) juices were returning to normal!

Andrew's natural brain wave was *his* visceral brain-wave controller. It controlled all of his visceral organs and kept them healthy, providing that he didn't abuse them with improper eating and living habits.

Andrew practiced to bring back his natural brain wave every time he ate—as well as *after* he ate. He gradually stopped belching after meals and, before long, his crawling headaches disappeared.

Overcoming Constipation Without Drugs (11 Secrets)

The long sitting postures of the Yogis contribute immensely to constipation. The hour-after-hour sessions of sitting with their hips flattened against the ground slows down abnormally the blood flow through their pelvis and solidifies the fecal matter drifting into their rectums. Here are the unfailing Yogi tricks to bring your constipation under your control:

1. The Yogis keep regular hours, and it helps them with their bowels. To train your own bowels to be regular, you have to urge them to move at approximately the same time every day. That alone, though, won't end your constipation.

2. You have to exercise (or contract) your abdominal muscles regularly. They initiate your peristaltic wave to drive the wastes in your alimentary tract along, through your colons, to your rectum for evacuation.

3. You have to eat food that contains bowel-moving roughage. Fruits and vegetables contain it. One scientific authority believes that the roughage of fruits and vegetables is not enough.[1] You also need, he insists, the roughage of cereals and whole grain wheat. Although I don't disagree with him entirely, too much cereal also tends to fatten your waist and ruin your figure. A couple mouthfuls of cereal a day is all you can afford to take and still retain your figure without dieting or exercising hard.

A more effective way which my medical and Yogi ancestors found, is to eat *two* different roughage-containing raw fruits, like oranges and apples, or oranges and pineapples, *at the same meal*. If one such food alone doesn't move your bowels regularly, two of them, eaten at the same meal, seem to trigger your bowels into action, and with regularity. Of all the natural roughages, indeed, we have found that the white of the orange skin is the most effective for bowel movement. Peel off thinly the yellow skin of the orange and leave on most of the white. Eject the seeds from the center of the orange, where they are massed. Drop the remainder of the orange in a fruit juicer or food grinder and let it chop up the white of the orange fine enough not to require too much mastication. You will be amazed at how effectively it will bring your constipation under control.

Caution: Eating plain oranges (even if ground up or finely chopped) sensitizes your teeth and attacks their enamel. Eat oranges with a banana and drink their juice through a straw.

4. Do Your Appetite Controller, page 53, to crush the fecal matter within your lower intestine. This Yoga mov-asana will fracture the fecal matter into smaller masses, so that it will resist much less the rectum-ward push of your peristaltic waves (the wave-like contractions of your alimentary tract which pulsate from your stomach to your rectum). Eat nothing between meals, or the mov-asana will trigger your peristaltic waves into action *before* there is enough waste matter in your lower colon for a full evacuation.

5. Eat very little of soft, white flour products. These foods create "brick hard" bowels. And drink from six to eight glasses of water a day to help your alimentary tract form fecal matter moist enough to be easily thrust rectal-ward by your peristaltic waves. (This is *plus* your food-time liquids.)

6. Avoid laxatives. Resort to enemas but once in several months, or longer, if you have to. Train your bowels to evacuate *naturally*, without artificial help. *Never force them*, or you will encourage them to form hemorrhoids.

7. At breakfast make it a practice to eat silently, if you expect your bowels to move shortly after you leave the table. Due to your interest in the conversation your taste glands will lose their intimate connection with your peristaltic wave and fail to trigger it into action. This is an *important prerequisite* to follow for successful, daily, after-breakfast bowel movement! The same rule applies to any regular bowel movement period you have trained yourself into.

8. Gas-producing foods, like figs, or even fig cookies, also stimulate regular bowel movements in you. Upon arising after a night's sleep, take one and one-half glasses of *very* warm water. Follow it, if your bowels are very obstinate, with sets of Your Appetite Controller, page 53, to force the walls of your stomach to try to compress the water. And since water is non-compressible, your stomach walls will be "stretched" instead and will burst into peristaltic waves in the attempt to compress the water.

9. Keep regular hours as much as possible to train your peristaltic waves to contract and dilate all the way down your alimentary canal at approximately the same time every day and synchronize with your biological clock.

10. Avoid long periods of sitting, whenever possible. If you cannot help it, try to be on your feet, or walk if you can, from seven to ten minutes every hour. If you have enough privacy, squeeze or massage your hips with your hands for at least two minutes at that time, to stimulate their circulation back to normal. This

applies equally when you are at home watching television, working at your hobby, or enjoying social life.

11. Except from during late afternoon until bedtime, don't let more than one and one-half hours elapse between your drinking water during the day (not counting meal time). Portions of your bowel matter, otherwise, will turn so hard and dry that they will form fecal plugs and constipate you, partially at least.

By faithfully observing these 11 simple but unfailing rules, you will swiftly bring your frustrating constipation under control. . . and *without drugs*.

A Simple Activity That Guarantees Regular Elimination, The Quadrops Yoga Mov-asana

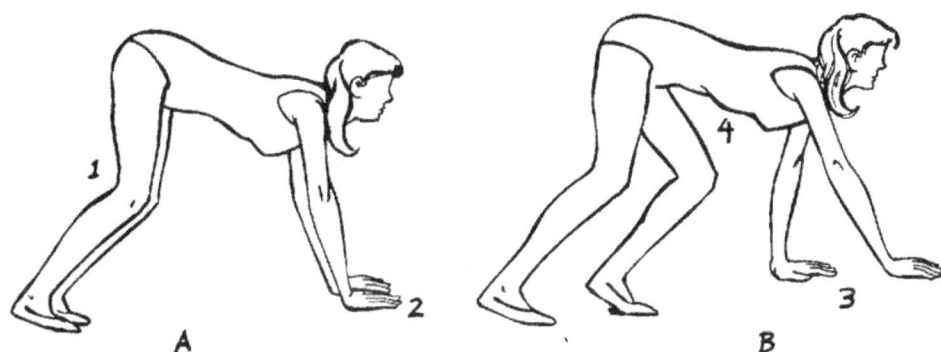

Figure 32
The Quadrops Yoga Mov-asana

The position to assume (Figure 32A)

1. Bend knees and place hands on floor.

How to do this Yoga mov-asana (Figure 32B)

2. Move hands far enough forward to gradually straighten your knees.

3. Walk across room on hands and feet, like an ape. With each step try to draw your feet closer to your hands. (Remember to do so gradually.)

4. Your waist will draw in so tightly that it will feel as if cramped. Visualize in that feeling your adrenal glands being crushed in your stomach (even though they are in your lower back).

5. Stand up again. All your rancor against the world will have vanished, and your circadian rhythms will alter to conform to your new self. When you face anyone with this frame of mind, his (or her) own circadian rhythms will alter to coincide with yours, and his (or her) own adrenals will be suppressed. He (or she) will consider *you* his most needed tranquilizer.

Frequency: 1 repetition. 1 set. 5 times a week.

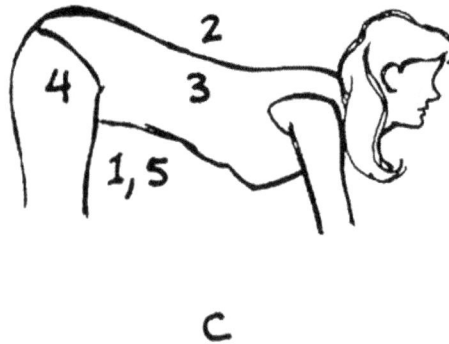

C

Figure 32, cont.

What The Quadrops Yoga mov-asana does for you (Figure 32C)

1. Draws in your waistline like a corset.

2. Temporarily places your back in the most healthy four-legged position for proper alignment of your vertebrae.

3. Helps to rejuvenate your back by stretching its compressed intervertebral discs and relieving them of your body weight.

4. The corset-like grip on your waist tends to regulate your peristaltic wave if you suffer from constipation.

5. Keeps your general waistline drawn in. Improves brain circulation.

How Alma T. Threw off Her Burden of Irregularity

For over 20 years Alma T. had been plagued with stubborn bowels. She had tried laxatives, enemas regularly, jogging, swimming and other exigencies. She had quit laxatives because she feared becoming an addict. But the other "things" worked too irregularly. Alma needed something more reliable to add to her food roughage and her fruits and vegetables.

I urged her to add a tablespoon of cereal to her diet, and to reduce it to half after several weeks. I also taught her The Quadrops mov-asana. It flattened her waist so firmly against the dry waste matter obstructing her lower colon that it broke it up for peristaltic response. When she stood erect, after The Quadrops position, her waistline felt as if drawn in by a girdle.

Next morning Alma's bowels moved easier than they had for some time. Within two weeks she forgot that she had even been constipated. Her waist was girlish now, too. Her desperate dream had come true.

Eliminating the Causes of Hemorrhoids

Since the Yogis sit for long periods of time, their buttocks are flattened by the hard ground, threatening them with constipation—and hemorrhoids. But they know how to combat these afflictions. My medical ancestors and I used these Yoga secrets on large numbers of people and enjoyed miraculous success with them. This is a simple Yogi way to eliminate hemorrhoids:

1. Peel a clove of garlic of about the length and thickness of the first third of your little finger. Scrape the sides of it with a sharp knife to expose its moisture. Spread your rectum open and insert most of the shaved garlic into it. Draw it out after from three to four seconds, no longer.

Within a half minute or less you will feel a "burning" within your rectum. Its mucous membrane lining is being constricted, and the hemorrhoidal vein in it is being shrunk.

Repeat this procedure for about three nights, just before going to bed. Repeat it more times if you have to, but most of the time one repetition is sufficient. Within a few days, even if you do it only once, you will note a decided difference in the size of the hemorrhoidal vein protrusion. It will soon disappear. Should it ever return, repeat the procedure.

A Wise Diet to Help Diminish Your Risks from Insecticides in Your Foods

In the laboratory, flooding the target cells of your body (say, your liver) with a diet supplemented with methionine, cystine, or casein, which can react with the insecticide AAF, will reduce the possibilities of your getting tumors from insecticides. (Discovered by James A. Miller and Elizabeth C. Miller of the McArdle Laboratory and confirmed by other scientists.) Methionine is found in whole egg, egg white, meat, fish, corn, casein, and wheat. Cystine is found in egg white and whole egg. Flooding the target cells of your body on weekends, in addition, with garlic helps avoid cancer because several sets of oxidizing enzymes are in greater concentration in your liver and kidneys than in the rest of your body. These enzymes, it is true, detoxify and dispose of foreign chemicals in your body. But they also activate the carcinogen (cancer-forming product). Flooding your body with chemicals that can react with the ultimate cancer-forming product will *inhibit* the reaction of the cancer-forming product within your cells. Garlic is an ideal chemical compound for achieving this because it can "donate" a methyl compound to the cancer-forming product (the carcinogen) either from the nitrogen or the sulphur atom in its molecule. So, eat regularly of the methionine and cystine containing foods during the week, but also include garlic in from one to three of your weekend meals. That is a wise diet to help diminish your cancer risks from insecticides in your food.

The Only Food to Keep Your Stomach Healthy Between Meals

Many different "light" foods and drinks are recommended to be taken between meals to keep up your strength, to prevent you from getting hungry, and the like. Even certain vitamins are taken between meals. Nearly 200 years of professional practice by my ancestors, plus my own lifetime of engaging in trials and experiments and my years of professional studies in medicine, dentistry, and chiropractic, have convinced me, without any element of a doubt, that the *only* between-meals food which keeps your stomach healthy is *water*.[2] Any other food stimulates a degree of digestion in your stomach between meals and brings on stomach acidity, and eventually stomach trouble. Even fruit juices stimulate digestion.

So, as soon as you feel hungry between meals, drink a glass, or a glass and one-half (if you feel very thirsty) of water. It will fill your stomach and vanquish the hunger. When you feel hungry again, drink more water. Do so until one hour before your next meal. (Eat three meals a day, unless your doctor or healer specifies otherwise). Try to drink water every hour, starting one and one-half hours after breakfast and lunch. But drink none for an hour before lunch and supper. And drink less water in the afternoon, and none after supper, so as not to have to frequent the urinal more than once or so after going to bed. You will be amazed at how different your stomach will soon feel.

Yoga Ways to Steer Clear of Diabetes

Diabetes is a particularly dangerous affliction because of its possible adverse complications. Among them are premature cataracts and possible hardening of the arteries. There is also a high incidence of kidney infection, and the lens of the eye swells, leading to its destruction. Certain proteins thicken and clog the filtering system of your kidneys and lead to uremia (or to backed up poison in your urine), a common cause of kidney death. The clogging is due to your high blood sugar and to your deficiency of insulin to absorb it out of your blood.

To steer clear of diabetes you should not often eat foods containing much sugar. You overwork your pancreas otherwise, until its insulin-producing glands wear out in exhaustion and can no longer synthesize enough of it to reduce the sugar content of your urine to normal. You should not go on fasts, either, or the insulin-producing glands of your pancreas (the Islands of Langerhans) will atrophy eventually from lack of enough use.[3]

Be pancreas-conscious, in other words. Eating sweets between meals, or gobbling down desserts at the end of your meal, or pouring too much sugar into, or on, whatever you drink at mealtime (or at any time), or indulging too regularly in candies, pastries, and other too-sweet foods, can lead to diabetes. To help you escape it, also do Your Appetite Controller (page 53), Your Diurnal Swing-Ho (page 85), and The Splanchnic Double Curl (page 162).

Yoga Secrets to Avoid Many Serious Diseases, Including Cancer of the Stomach, Intestines, Colon and Rectum

To possess an hourglass figure you have to eat small meals with little bulk. But such a diet, as I taught and published as early as 1954[4], and repeated in print in 1969[5], slows down the speed of the transit of your digesting food through your alimentary tract, thereby contributing to constipation, hemorrhoids, and other related digestive ills. Science made this same discovery *20 years later*.[6] Added to the list of ills are, in fact, among others, cancer of the colon or rectum, intestinal polyps (a type of benign growth), diverticular diseases, and heart disease. Permitting food wastes to stagnate too long in the alimentary tract, in brief, is truly dangerous. My students and readers who followed my 1954 Yoga secrets discovery (and diet), greatly minimized (if not got rid of) their perils of falling victim to such tragic maladies. People who did not learn about it until 1974 from science, risked joining (and many probably did join) the alarming percentage of the population who suffer from such killers today.

Science's suggested "important defense" against these death-dealing illnesses is to add bulk (fiber) to your diet. . . or *exactly* what I myself prescribed in my *Solar Diet* 20 years before. Today's science, also as I did 20 years before, recommends for bulk vegetables and fruits, such as: broccoli, Brussel sprouts, cabbage, beets, carrots, sweet potatoes, berries, tomatoes, eggplant, summer squash. I go even further, like the Yogis, and recommend turnips, apples, and oranges eaten together with the whites of the oranges unpeeled,[7] cauliflower, endive, beans, pineapple, mangoes, papaya, and many other tropical, sub-tropical, and temperate foods.

Science, too, agrees now with my statement of 1954[8] that cereal is very effective against these sicknesses. Science, in fact, considers cereal the most effective of all the bulk foods.[9] But I insist that the starch in cereal will add too much weight to your body, unless you consume no more than a heaping teaspoonful (at most) of it a day. (Science will prove me to be right again, as it has done so frequently.) Science, indeed, recommends bran, particularly after it is separated from the cereal.[10] But, 20 years ago I already warned *against* eating separated bran. I pointed out that it scrubbed too drastically the lining of the alimentary tract, and urged my students and readers to eat only the foods which still had the bran on them, such as whole grains. I repeat the warning, 20 years later and predict that science, once more, will discover me to be again correct. Separated bran, I insist, can lead to stomach ulcers, as well as to cancer of the colon—and possibly of the rectum. Bran also dehydrates your system, over-thickening your blood and straining your kidneys. Food with bulk, nonetheless, is a sure way to avoid many serious diseases (including cancer) of the stomach, intestines, colon, and rectum, and also appendicitis, polyps, and diverticulosis.

Another important reason against too much cereal is that it contains too much phytic acid. Like oxalic acid (found in prunes, cranberries, tomatoes, rhubarb, and spinach), it robs your bones of calcium, which can cause them to soften as you grow older, and the excreted phytic salt can irritate your bladder and perhaps eventually cause cystic cancer. Except for the cereal, your bulky foods should be eaten raw, that is, shredded, grated, or ground (grain). If cooked, the bulk food will also constipate you.

The Secret Right-Size of a Healthy Waistline

The common belief in the West is that the healthy waistline is that of the hourglass figure. For thousands of years the Yogis have known better. When you eat a filling meal (skimpy meals are de-energizing and constipating) containing sufficient bulk food, your waistline won't look as small until the food is digested as when you eat unhealthy, cancer-forming small meals with little bulk. Bulk retains water as it passes through your digestive tract. It thereby prevents your bowels from forming hard, dry masses that constipate you, transit slowly through you, irritate the lining of your digestive tract and threaten it with ulcers or cancer. Bulk also creates a certain quantity of gas which stimulates your peristaltic wave to drive your food onwards. But the retained water and the gas add volume to the digesting mass in your stomach and intestines and distend your waistline from one to two inches more than when you eat food with little bulk. The size of your waistline then, however, is your *healthy*, *right-sized waistline* for from two to three hours following the meal.

Should you constrict it with a tight belt, girdle, or any other kind of clothing to retain your smallest waist measurement after a healthy meal with bulk-food, you bring on indigestion, ruin your liver and pancreas, and burden your heart by forcing the gas created by your bulk-food up against it. Cramped for room, your crowded heart is compelled to pump more vigorously and strain itself unnecessarily. Drinking water between meals, too, as you are directed to in another section, keeps your waistline regularly distended another inch or so. But your stomach and intestines are intended to digest your food and replenish your lost energy. They are not expected to remain flat and half-empty all day, so you can "appear" always wasp-waisted at the risk of developing cancer as you grow older. They are supposed to expand, like an animal after it eats.

Your waist will still look its normal size once your stomach is empty again, an hour or more before your next meal. The rest of the time, though, it will be providing you with the energy and enthusiasm of youth.

If you are a man, for that reason, stop wearing unhealthy, liver-strangling belts and change to suspenders. If you are a woman, stop wearing girdles or other garments which fit your torso like straight-jackets and impede its freedom of movement. Liberate yourself from the tortures of styles which only cripple you and speed you to an early grave. That is an important Yoga secret for extraordinary health and a long life. Adopt it, as the Yogis did.

References

[1]Dr. Denis P. Burlitt, member of the British Medical Research Council's external scientific staff.

[2]Frank Rudolph Young, *Solar Diet* (West Nyack, N.Y.: Parker Publishing Company, Inc., 1954), p. 23.

[3]*Ibid.*, p. 16.

[4]*Ibid.*, p. 16.

[5]Frank Rudolph Young, *Yoga For Men Only* (West Nyack, N.Y.: Parker Publishing Company, Inc., 1969), p. 179.

[6]*Reader's Digest*, December 1974, p. 105.

[7]Frank Rudolph Young, *Somo-Psychic Power: Using Its Miracle Forces for a Fabulous New Life* (West Nyack, N.Y.: Parker Publishing Company, Inc., 1974), p. 173.

[8]*Reader's Digest*, December 1974, p. 105.

[9]*Ibid.*

[10]*Ibid.*

10

How Yoga Renews
Sexual Attractiveness

How You Lose Your Sexual Attractiveness

Those who cannot control their sex drives and habitually pursue different prospects for sex, or even their mates for excessive sex, become no better—or worse—than chronic masturbators. The only difference is that the chronic masturbator lacks the social boldness to convert his sex fantasies into realities.

Sex partners who cannot control their drives also tend to squander their prime time and energy in an activity which promises no permanent value or long-lasting return. Once they reach the climax, their ecstacy is over, and the post-coital conversation degenerates into monotony or hypocrisy. Each partner then feels that the conquest has been achieved. It is time now to clean up the used parts and return to reality.

Anyone who is a chronic masturbator or an abnormal sex-chaser regularly wastes his physical voltage and keeps his physical and mental vitality under par. Whether you are male or female, you can learn the Yoga secret to stop wasting your physical voltage and acquire the sex energy of the superman and the bewitching pull of the desired woman.

How a Yoga Secret Stops Wasting Your Physical Voltage

Of course most Yogis left sex behind as they withdrew from the material world. Certain of them, however, employed a well-guarded secret to multiply their sex energies without vitamins, hormones, or other artificial means. The Yogis who rejoined the material world discovered that this secret increased their physical voltage, giving them more massive erections, multiplying their copulation time, and providing them with a natural method of birth control. This secret freed these Yogis from sexual enslavement by others and helped them retain their sexual energies so that they suffered comparatively little after-sex fatigue.

The simple explanation of this secret I base upon the extensive knowledge and professional investigation of my medical ancestors, plus my own experience in chiropractic. Your pubic hair, whether you are a man or a woman, multiplies genital heat (crotch or pelvic heat). The multiplied heat can overexcite sex glands because it penetrates deep into their adjoining tissues. It can convert a controlled individual into a sexual-activity slave or a masturbation addict, draining off nerve-electricity.

To protect yourself against this wasteful sapping of your physical voltage, shave off your pubic hair once a month! You will be TRULY LIBERATED then! You will be released from the insatiable sexual mania which may leave your nerve endings tender (particularly those of your thighs, so that your thighs suffer from sudden contractions or tics), your cheeks deeply hollowed, and yourself nervous, anxious, generally debilitated, and readily subject to fatigue (especially if you are a man). This insatiable sexual mania depletes your physical vitality, as well as your hidden mental and physical powers. Mystics and professional strong men conserve their semen-energy (semergy, see *Yoga For Men Only*[1]) and convert themselves into supermen in performing miracles or in muscle power. They would become pulps of erectile tissue otherwise, with strained prostates and sponge-like minds and bodies.

Secret of Magic Sex Power

Last but not least, as a sex aid for a man, shaving off pubic hairs permits sex organ to enlarge more during sexual intercourse. This is because no significant amount of crotch heat is drained off into his mate through interlocking pelvic hairs. When both partners have shaved their pubic hair, in addition, they can easily avoid falling victim to the mutually disappointing "quickie" orgasm. A man can delay orgasm for hours—or even prevent it altogether while his mate experiences several.

Yogis who rejoined the material world have maintained erections for eight hours of rather continuous copulation. They withdrew several times for short rests without ejaculation, and resumed a few minutes later with full potency. Two of them withheld debilitating orgasms for years, while triggering hundreds of them in their mates. The Yogi secret of fantastic sex-energy retention is an ideal natural method for birth control, besides, without the use of pills or contraceptives. It offends no religion and brings on no dangerous side effects.

If you fear cutting yourself while shaving your pubic hair, slip a comb through the hair and clip it off with a scissors, the way a barber cuts hair. But even if you shave it off, don't try to shave it clean to the skin. Leave a quarter-inch of hair; otherwise stubs from the opposite sides of your body could meet when you close your legs and itch you. But don't let the hair grow back longer than three-quarters of an inch, or it will multiply your genital (pelvic) heat. Keep your pubic region shaved close enough, and you will automatically increase your physical voltage and turn into a superman with fantastic sex-energy retention. You will be unsurpassed as a lover! If you are a woman, it will save you from being a passion slave at the mercy of false men.

An Optic Brain Wave That Results in Charming Eyes
(No figure necessary.)

1. Sit in a chair, facing the mirror.

2. Imagine that your image is the person you want.

3. Recall vividly how you feel whenever you meet him (or her), whether on the street, in the office, on a date, or in any other situation. Then ask yourself *honestly*: Do you feel
    (a) Frightened?
    (b) Excited?
    (c) Uncertain of yourself?
    (d) Skeptical?
    (e) Frustrated?
    (f) Overeager?
    (h) Disgusted and ashamed?
    (i) Bewildered?

4. However you feel, your brain will create its own natural brain waves to fit *your own* state of mind. You don't have to record these brain waves or test them on a biofeedback device to know what they are. *Everybody's brain waves are different for the same emotion.* In some people, alpha brain waves affect them like *theta* waves. In other people, theta brain waves affect them like alpha. There is no *proven brain wave state* measurement for everybody. The most accurate brain wave for you to adopt is *the one you radiate during the very situation it is produced*.

So, relive *the* situation that troubles you and note *exactly how you feel* during it.

5. Think, next, of how you *would* feel if you could draw to you the mate you want *at a glance*.

6. Practice this several times, until *that new brain wave* is *yours. That* is the right optic brain wave to excite instantly the person you want, because it will exude out of your eyes when you use it. And your eyes will turn enchanting at a glance.

Recharging Yourself with Potency
Through Oriental Hip Mov-asana

You can recharge yourself sexually for greater vim and potency with the Oriental Hip mov-asana. Here is how to do it. (Follow Figure 33.)

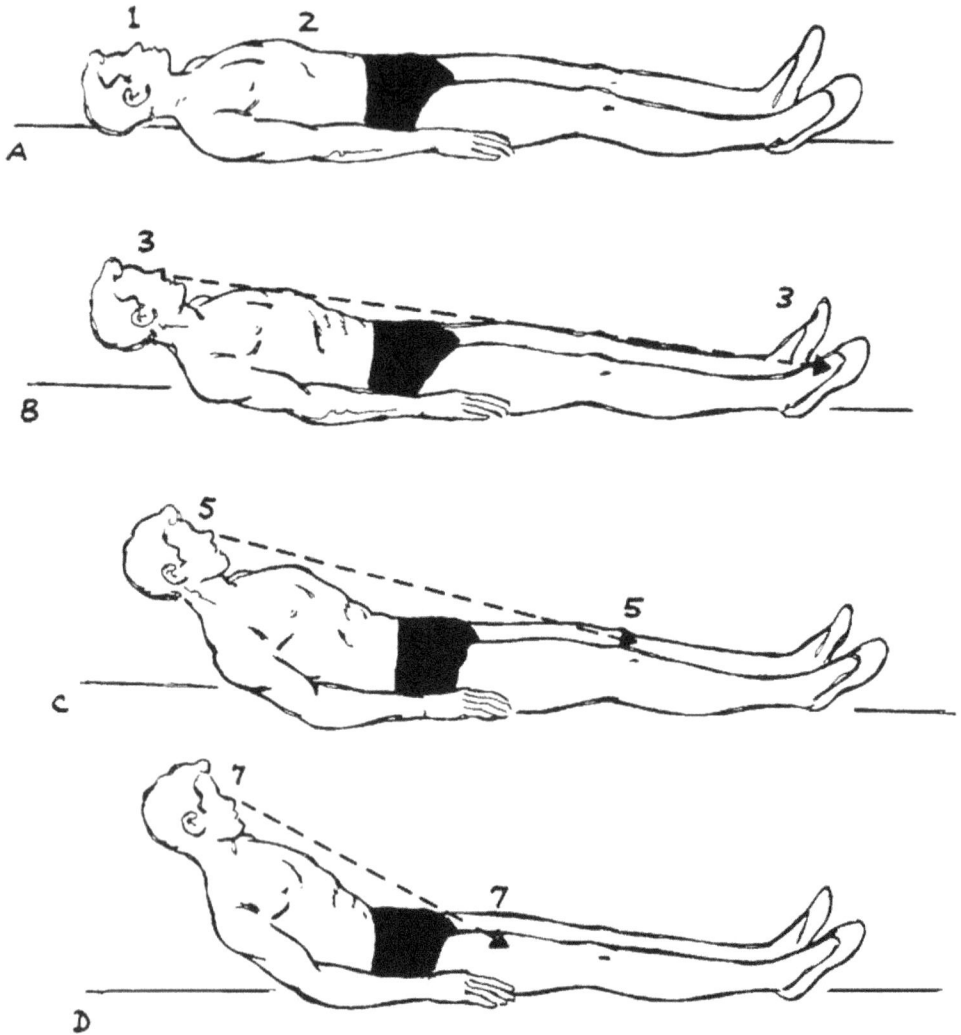

Figure 33
Oriental Hip Mov-asana

The position to assume (Figure 33A)

1. Lie flat on your back on your bed or floor, with

2. Arms extended along your sides, or on your thighs.

How to do this Yoga mov-asana (Figures 33B,C,D)

3. Raise your head and try to see the floor between your *feet* (Figure 33B).

4. Repeat three times. Then rest about one-half minute. Now,

5. Raise your head higher and try to see the floor between your *knees* (Figure 38C).

6. Also repeat this three times. Rest another one-half minute. Finally,

7. Raise your head very high and try to see the floor between your *thighs* (Figure 39D).

8. Also repeat this three times. That constitutes one set.

Frequency: 2 sets. 3 or 4 times a week.

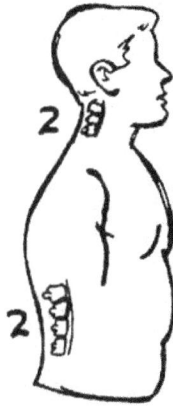

Figure 33, cont.

What The Oriental Hip mov-asana does for you (Figure 33E)

1. Flattens the upper half of your waist, the "pork belly" part, which bulges easily.

2. Stimulates the vertebrae of your lower back (your 1-4 lumbars), and of the lower half of your neck (your 3-7 cervicals). Thus, it improves your uterus (if you are a woman), bladder, liver, diaphragm. If you are a man, it excites the sympathetics to your penis and your pudendal nerve, drawing more blood to the organ and more easily exciting an erection. By keeping your legs close together when doing it, too, it increases your crotch heat and recharges your potency even faster.

How To Contact Your Past Lives with The Oriental Hip mov-asana (No Figure)

1. Lie in bed after completing the mov-asana and *wish fervently* to contact your *last* past life, or whichever past one you wish.

2. Feel your whole body "come together" into one microscopic bullet. Shoot this bullet into a sperm or ovum in your sex glands and let it saturate itself with it. Your sperm or ovum (egg) contains your genes, and your genes carry the inherited pattern of your past lives. Visualize yourself contacting the particular past life which you want to contact most. Different genes in your sperm or ovum inherit different lives from your different ancestors. If you contact the wrong one, your microscopic bullet will withdraw from it swiftly and shoot into another until it finds the right one. It might have to shoot into several different genes before it contacts the right one.

3. When it does you will feel so much at home in that past life that you will "separate" from your present one. Your physiological rhythm will alter to harmonize with it. With a little practice you will soon astonish yourself with your ability to contact any past life of yours that you want to. The secret is developed still more in the case history which follows.

How Marilyn D. Contacted a Past Life of Hers and Extracted Sex-Enslaving Secrets

Marilyn D. was deeply disappointed with her marriage. So was her husband, John. In desperation Marilyn read books about sex techniques and applied them in their love-making. John enjoyed the different ones at first, but soon wearied of them. They were too practiced and outright for him. Marilyn wondered whether some past female ancestor of hers had been a sexual bewitcher, and if she could appeal to her for help.

I taught Marilyn The Oriental Hip Mov-asana to recharge herself. It drew in her abdomen tightly and squeezed it into veritable nothingness. Marilyn released trapped gas and felt more limber at once. At the end of the sets she appeared noticeably trimmer already, felt lighter around the waist, and lost much of the discomfort in her right side.

After doing it for two weeks and beautifying her waist and breasts remarkably, Marilyn tried to contact a past life of hers in which she might have had a sexual bewitcher as a close relative. She felt her whole body turn into a microscopic bullet, and after several minutes of shooting different ovums in her ovary, she felt it enter one which "separated" her from her present existence. Her physiological rhythms blended with it, and she completely forgot her present existence and *lived* in her past one.

Before Marilyn's very eyes, it seemed, an enchantress appeared who bore a distant resemblance to her aunt. The enchantress spoke to her like an interested sister and confided to her amazing secrets of how to fascinate men.

When Marilyn "returned to earth" she was an entirely different person romantically. Her husband was blindly smitten with her. Over the months he showered her with presents and took her, as "rewards," to one thrilling vacation spot after another.

The Remarkable Effects of Yoga Knee Bends on Sex Energy

The Torso Push (page 36), The Sacro-Stretch (page 201), and Your Easy Hip Trimmer (page 58) bring considerable amounts of blood to your pelvic region to supply the muscles of your thighs and hips. Like all your skeletal muscles, the blood supply to your thighs and hips is augmented by your sympathetic nervous system. This same nervous system supplies your ovaries (if you are a woman) or your testicles (if you are a man). Since your ovaries or testicles are also located in your pelvic area, they, too, are unusually supplied with blood when you do these mov-asanas, and their sex-energy production is increased. When you do these mov-asanas with enough regularity, your sex glands are increased regularly and permanently. That's why Yoga knee bends exert remarkable effects on your sex-energy.

Increasing Your Sex Appeal with Yoga Mov-asanas

The Pectoral 90 Yoga mov-asana is the well-guarded Yoga secret for giving you fantastic sex appeal. Here is how to do it (Follow Figure 34.)

The position to assume (Figure 34A)

1. Stand close to a table, bedstead, sink, or anything strong enough to resist your push,
2. Feet normally hip-width (about 8 inches) apart. Don old gloves.
3. Cup fingers (palms forwards) against edge of table.
4. Use a very wide grip. Space each hand about 12 inches outside each shoulder.

How to do this Yoga mov-asana (Figure 34B)

1. Inhale deeply, straightening or arching your back. (Not shown).
2. Press hard with your fingers against the edge of the table.
3. Resist them with your body, mainly by locking your hips, knees, and spine, as much as necessary.
4. Continue pressing with your fingers until your body bends over completely against the resistance of your fingers. But,

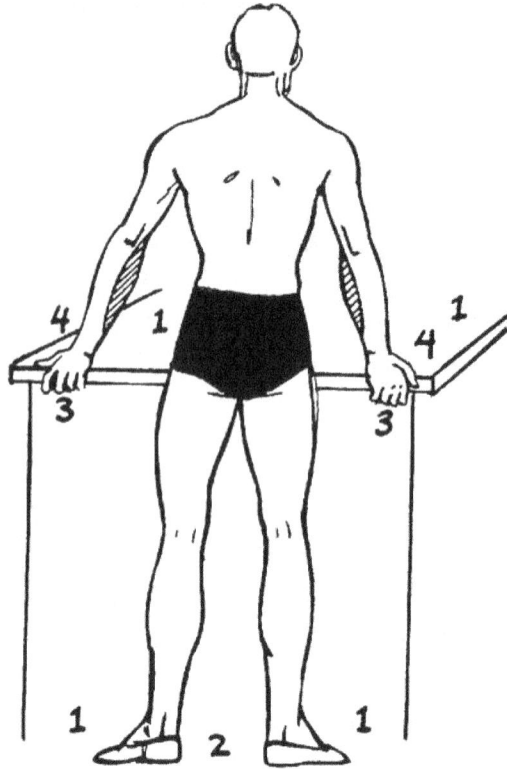

A

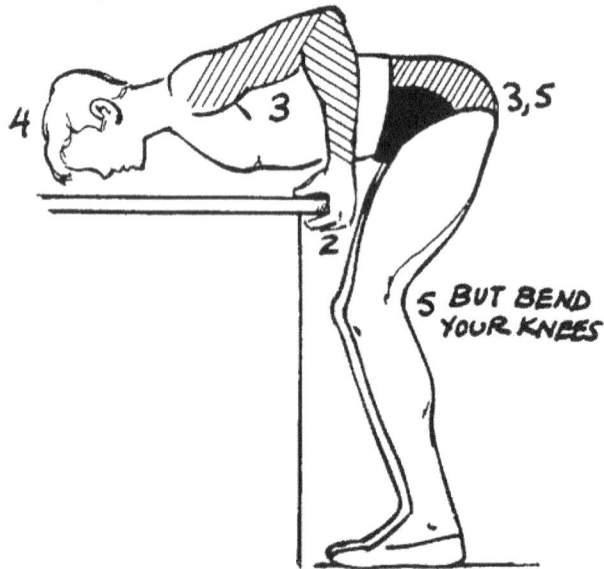

B
Figure 34
The Pectoral 90 Yoga Mov-asana

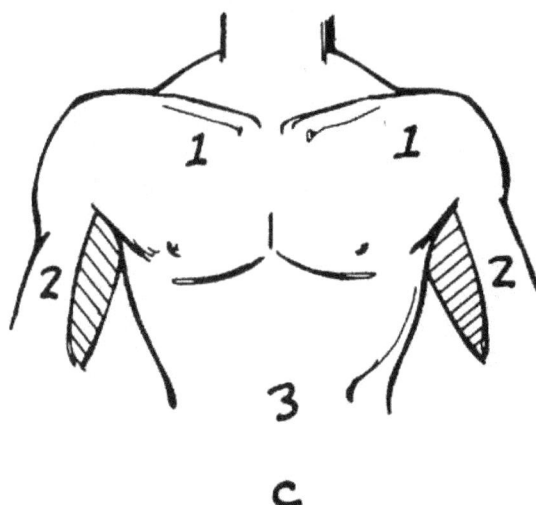

C

Figure 34, cont.

5. As your body bends over, *bend your knees* slightly, and draw in your hips a little.

Frequency: 5 repetitions. 2 sets (groups of repetitions). 3 times a week.

What The Pectoral 90 mov-asana does for you:

1. Proportions the fronts of your shoulders and erases the bony look. It is *fantastic* for this. (With full power, if you are a man, makes your shoulders massive. With medium force, if you are a woman, makes your shoulders elegant and girlish).

2. Proportions the fronts of your arms to restore your toned-up youthful look and erase the "droopy arm look" of middle age and older.*

*Particularly if, during the simple movement, you keep your forearms nearly perpendicular to the table. With full strength, if you are a man, gives you enormous biceps. With medium force, if you are a woman, trims but firms your arms.

3. Draws in your waistline considerably when you bend your knees and draw in your hips.

4. Stimulates the vertebrae of your upper middle back (your 4-5 dorsals), and the one close to the base of your spine (your 4 lumbar). Your aorta and heart improve. The visceral spasms of the farther end of your stomach, and of your duodenum (small intestine) and lower bowel (colon) relax.

5. Alters your pessimistic outlook to an optimistic one.

How Orland B. Got the Girl He Wanted

Orland B. lived in virtual misery. He was insanely in love with a "stunner," as he described her. But she wouldn't give him a tumble, he grieved. Suitors flocked around her, but he himself seemed to hold no fascination for her. He lacked the "psychological vigor," he added, to be a raving success at anything. He lacked the "energy of tongue," the "go-getting physiology," so he had lost interest in life.

I taught Orland The Pectoral 90. It tightened his abdominal muscles, drew in his waistline and relaxed the visceral spasms of the farther end of his stomach. The fronts of his shoulders and arms brimmed with power, leaving him feeling capable of attaining anything he wanted to.

Reflexly, it filled him with a body-mind vigor which he had never suspected he had. His tongue grew loose, and he itched to bring others under his control. His digestion improved remarkably, and his bowels moved much better.

His "stunner," he noticed, observed him now as if for the first time. Other women noticed him keenly, too! To Orland's amazement, even the "stunner" was competing for him! Since *she* was the one he wanted most of all, Orland lost no time going after her and making her his bride.

That wasn't all! His commissions, over the months, actually multiplied! And the more he made, the more his physiological vigor increased. Within two years, his commissions rose to an incredible $55,000 a year, and were still climbing strong.

The Yoga Way to Create Your Own "Private Tissue" Fountain of Youth

Climbing to the top in life, whether you are a man or a woman, is not dangerous to your heart. I preached this as early as the 1930's when it was universally believed (and is still believed by many die-hards) that the tension of rising in life will shorten your life by bringing on, or leaving you prone to, a heart attack. A number of scientific studies in the last few years, however, have found that heart attack is *not* greatly influenced by the tensions of getting ahead in business.[2] Many have blamed it more on body-build, smoking and eating habits, social and educational background. Executives, indeed, suffer *less* from heart attacks than others in business! Men who are promoted rapidly, either frequently or recently, as well as men who are transferred to new departments or new companies, have no added risk of heart attack!

Executives and college students, in fact, had fewer seizures than other employees![3] The work stress on workers and non-college men, after all, is no less intense than for executives and college men. Workers and non-college workers deal with superiors, with noisy and dangerous machinery, with countless hazards of common work, and with the constant threat of the job coming to an unexpected end. Being an executive with the authority to fire a worker is no more stressful!

To create your own "private tissue" fountain of youth, you have to enjoy your work. You have to lose the baseless terror of driving yourself to an early grave just because your goals are high, or because you might "over-exercise," or because you are "getting old." Even if your work is not what you prefer, make yourself enjoy it until it is changed.

DO NOT try to trim your weight down to the gaunt stage. Athletes do so to try to acquire eye-gripping definition of their muscles. With fad diets, women shrink to wasp-like narrowness at their waists. But in both instances, too much submucous fat is melted off the body and face, contributing to premature wrinkling and the loss of the youthful look.

Last but not least, stay composed in the midst of pressure, whether it is daily or long-term. Assume the will to live long and healthily, and do the Yoga mov-asanas regularly.

References

[1]Frank Rudolph Young, *Yoga For Men Only* (West Nyack, N.Y.: Parker Publishing Company, Inc., 1971).

[2] A five-year study among Bell System employees conducted by Cornell University Medical College, New York, New York.

[3]*Ibid*.

11

Yoga Secrets

That Sharpen Your Mind

Unlocking Your Utmost Keenness of Mind

Your brain cells tire after two to four hours' use. They rest by daydreaming (responding to your inner stimuli) for one to two hours before regaining their energy to think effectively again (or to respond to your *external* stimuli). Your brain cells have alternations, in other words, which allow them to think, and then to shut off the noises of the world as they retire into daydreaming to digest your thoughts. That's why you seem to "grow dull" after long concentration. It is due to the circadian (daily) rhythms in the levels of important biochemicals (like epinephrine) in your brain.

To trigger your utmost keenness of mind, then, you have to control the secretion of epinephrine from your adrenal glands into your brain, so that your brain can remain at attention when it is time for it to grow dull. Your brain will then think *at its best pace any time you want it to*. A super-mind is primarily a "mistake-less" thinker. By making the fewest mistakes in its thinking, such a mind achieves the most for its efforts. It makes the fewest mistakes when it absorbs all the facts it is fed while at full attention, before retiring into itself, or into daydreaming, to digest them. The Yoga mov-asana to control the secretion of epinephrine from your adrenal glands into your brain and unlock your utmost keenness of mind, is Your Super-Mind Awakener. Here is how to do it. (Follow Figure 35.)

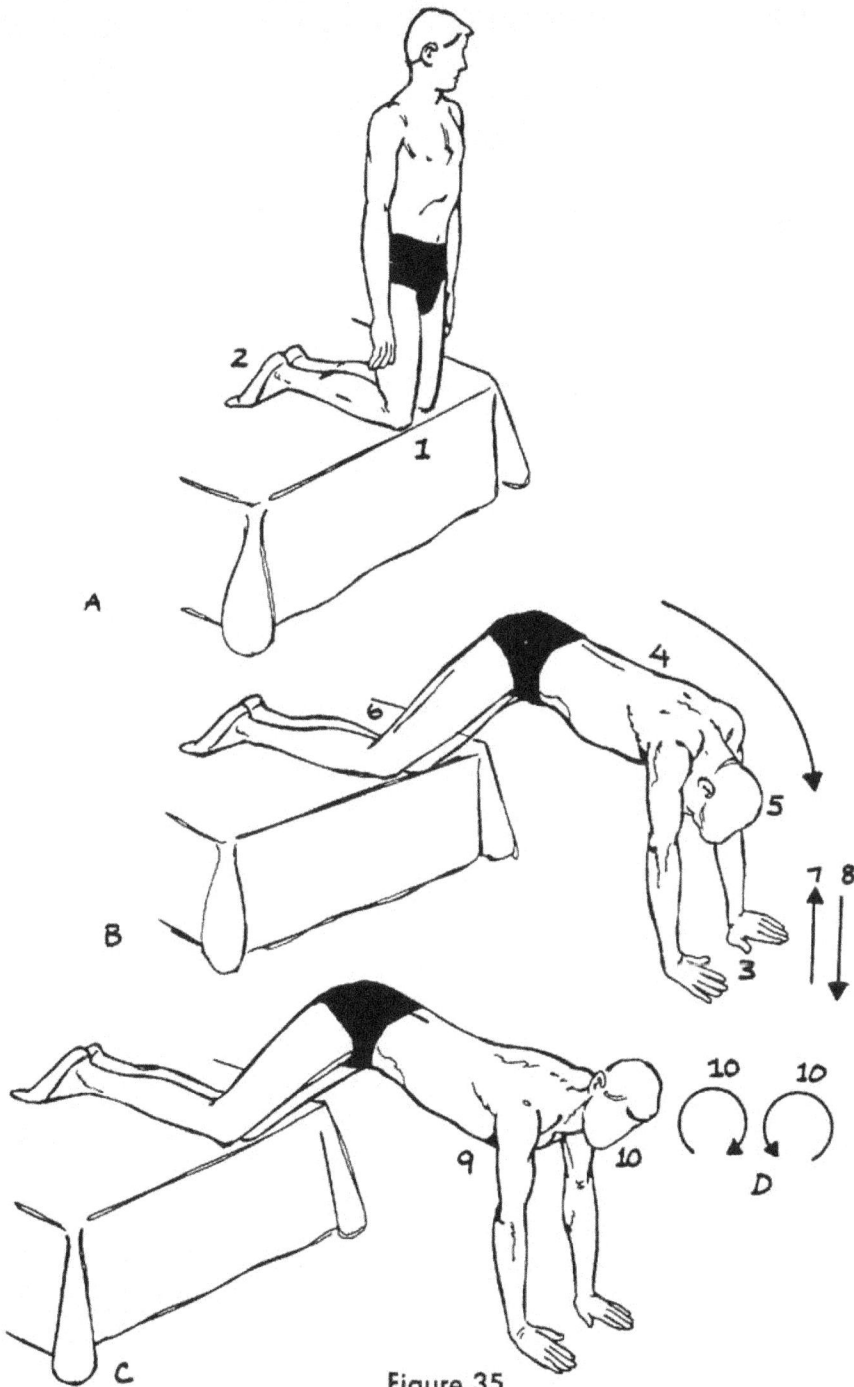

Figure 35
Your Super-Mind Awakener

The position to assume (Figure 35A)

    1. Kneel close to the edge of your bed,

    2. With your legs at right angles away from the edge.

How to do this Yoga mov-asana (Figures 35 B,D)

    3. Place your hands on the ground,

    4. With your body arched, and

    5. Your head down.

    6. Your calves and feet remain on the bed. Now,

    7. Raise your neck. Then lower it again. Do so ten times.

    8. Resume the position of Figure 35A to rest your hands and arms from supporting your overhanging torso.

    9. Then reassume the position of Figure 35B and

    10. Rotate your head five times in one direction, and five times in the other. (Figures 35 C,D).

What Your Super-Mind Awakener does for you:

    1. Flushes your brain with fresh blood, and washes away the old stagnating blood. It thereby supplies your brain with much more oxygen. Since oxygen is the major nutrient of your brain, it enables your brain to function at its best.

How Gilbert S. Suddenly Acquired a Miracle-like Mind

    Gilbert S. wondered how *I*, with my mind alone, without even a "true" laboratory, could make *scores* of the *most advanced* psychic discoveries from one to 36 years *ahead* of the leading scientists behind the Iron Curtain, with all their mammoth resources. How I even plucked their *exact scientific explanations* out of my sleeping super-mind.[2]

    I taught Gilbert his Super-Mind Awakener. This was one of the most important super-genius stimulators I used when trying to "pluck" ideas far-ahead-of-my-time, out of my sleeping super-mind—a mind which everybody has.

    When Gilbert tried it, fresh new blood flushed into his brain and washed away the stagnating old blood. At once his head felt clear and forceful. Its weariness was replaced by an indomitable eagerness to solve *any* problem, no matter how difficult. He leaped into the core of his problems and fearlessly cut a swath through them. To his own amazement, one solution after another which had totally eluded him before, dawned on him.

Gilbert retained that attitude for hours at first. Later, he retained it all day, and even after work. His mind was working like a miracle. Astounding opportunities for advancement opened to him which he had never dreamed of before.

A Yogi's Daily Psychic Power Trigger

Your pineal gland is located inside your head, close to the root of your nose. It is known as your psychic power gland. When you perform psychic feats you handle invisible forces and manifest them into form. But your hypothalamus, a nerve mass at the base of your brain, inhibits your pineal gland. So does stress. For your pineal gland, your psychic power gland, to function powerfully, you have to inhibit both your hypothalamus and your stress. To inhibit them you have to block all messages flashing from your brain, muscles, organs, and tissues to your hypothalamus. Although that is impossible, you can achieve it to a marked degree by *super-tranquilizing* yourself. Do so with the secret Yoga mov-asana, Your Daily ESP Trigger. This is how to do it. (Follow Figure 36.)

The position to assume (Figure 36A)

1. Write on a piece of paper the name of the person you want to win, or the goal you wish to achieve.

2. Lie on your bed without a pillow, flat on your back.

3. Place the piece of paper with the name or goal beneath your head.

How to do this Yoga mov-asana

4. The back of your head possesses eight times more nerve-electricity power than the front. Therefore,

5. Concentrate now on the piece of paper. Visualize clearly what you wrote on it. At the same time,

6. Press your head down hard upon the paper, and drive the full power of your nerve-electricity into it. Feel the muscles in the back of your neck turn firm (Figure 36B).

7. But hold the muscle contraction no longer than an instant.

8. Repeat. With each repetition, though, feel more and more nerve-electricity pour out of the back of your head into that paper, and visualize what

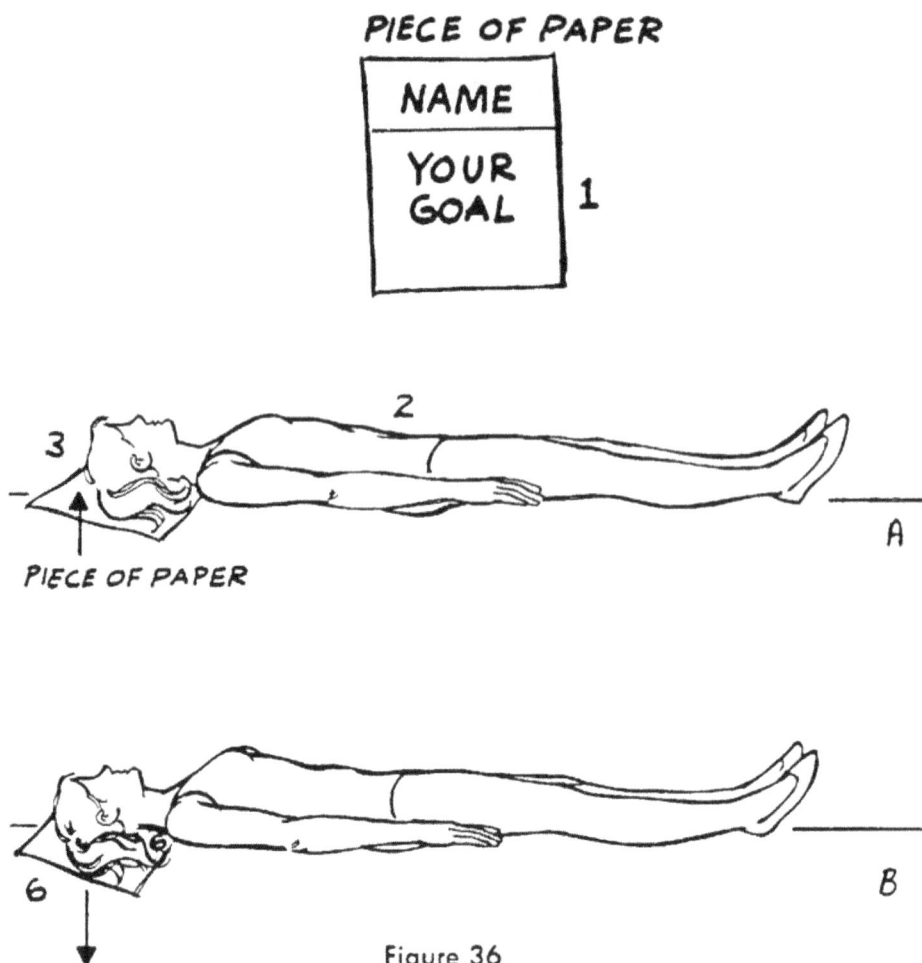

PIECE OF PAPER

Figure 36
Your Daily ESP Trigger

you wrote on it coming *100 percent true*, no less!

Frequency: 2 repetitions. 1 set (groups of repetitions). Do it every morning when you want to switch on your highest ESP potential.

What Your Daily ESP Trigger does for you (Figure 36 C):

1. Proportions wonderfully the back of your neck. If you are a woman, and don't press your head down with full force, it will reward you with a smooth, girlish neck.

2. Flushes more blood (with feeding oxygen) into your brain.

3. Implants what you wrote on paper firmly in your conscious and subconscious minds. (Also in your psychic power center in your forehead and temples areas, through association fibers which connect different areas of your brain to other areas of it.)

4. Leaves you feeling as tranquilized as if self-hypnotized. All stress has left you, thus blocking off the intensity of the messages flashed from your brain, muscles, organs, and tissues to your hypothalamus. Your pineal gland, your psychic power gland, is freed to function powerfully.

5. If you do Your Daily ESP Trigger upon arising, already before you start out every day you will switch on your full psychic power potentials and convert yourself swiftly into *the specific kind of person you wish to be that day*.

6. When you face the world that day, drive that accumulated super-amount of nerve-electricity out of your head *from any direction you wish*, at the most appropriate time. Your psychic power will dart out of it and dominate the situation, and make your worthy dreams come true.

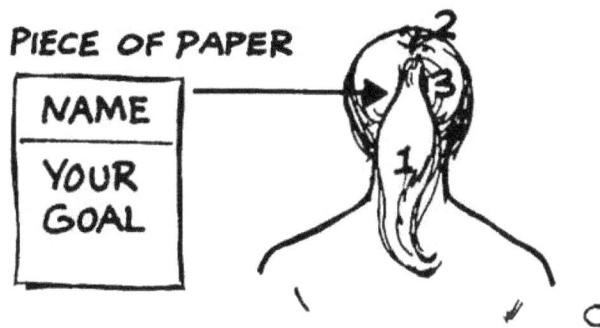

Figure 36, cont.

How Cleo R. Acquired Unusual Mental (Psychic) Power

Cleo R. was dissatisfied with the lines forming around her neck. She was not old enough to have them, she grieved; yet, they were deepening fast and spoiling her appearance.

I instructed Cleo to look straight ahead when she walked and keep her head up, instead of habitually staring at the ground, as if looking for coins. The village women of India walked with their heads straight for several miles a day, balancing loads on them. Their necks remained amazingly smooth.

Next, I taught Cleo Her Daily Morning ESP trigger. When she pressed the back of her head down upon the paper with each repetition, her neck muscles firmed and smoothed out the forming encircling wrinkles. It also helped Cleo walk with her head straight. As an extra reward, the mov-asana triggered unusual psychic power in her to project in any direction and dominate difficult daily situations with an ease she never dreamed possible. I accepted her for advanced psychic study.

How to Make Your Mind Seethe with Profitable Originality

Your emotions can accentuate or minimize the message of a hunch you get until it loses all resemblance to the original. If you are gripped with fear when you receive a practical hunch, your fear might fill you with too much caution to gain from it. If you are seized with anger, you might appraise the hunch with hostility and also fail to gain from it. Overcome this handicap and let the hunch permeate you and enable you to gain the most from it.

Your nervous system can be conditioned (taught new habits). Different life events may "teach" your blood vessels to constrict, or your pulse to race. The extent of this physiological learning in you also depends upon your biological time of day.

For you to "feel" something before it happens, then, you have to prevent your volcanic emotions from blinding you to the hunch at the time of day you receive it. You have to prevent them from throwing your circadian rhythms "out of beat" when they could be "in beat." The secret Yoga mov-asana to achieve this end is Your Emotion Ouster. This is how to do it. (Follow Figure 37.)

The Marvel of Your Emotion Ouster Mov-asana

The position to assume (Figures 37 A,B)

1. Place two chairs together (Figure 37 A).

2. Stand about 15 inches from their seats, if you are around six feet tall. Stand closer if you are shorter, and farther away if you are taller.

3. Rest both hands close to the edge of the seats, with your fingers pointing towards the back of the chairs. Start with a wide grip, with each hand one inch beyond the width of its corresponding shoulder. (Wear protective gloves.)

4. Bend knees and drop body weight upon hands.

5. Keep forearms perpendicular to the chair seats, and

6. Bend body forward and downward, so that

7. Your elbows bend about halfway (at right angles). Keep them drawn *inwards* (or towards your body).

8. Reassume your positions in Numbers 2 and 3 once more. But, now, round your shoulders (turn them inwards, downwards and backwards) *before* resting your hands on the chair seats (Figure 37 C).

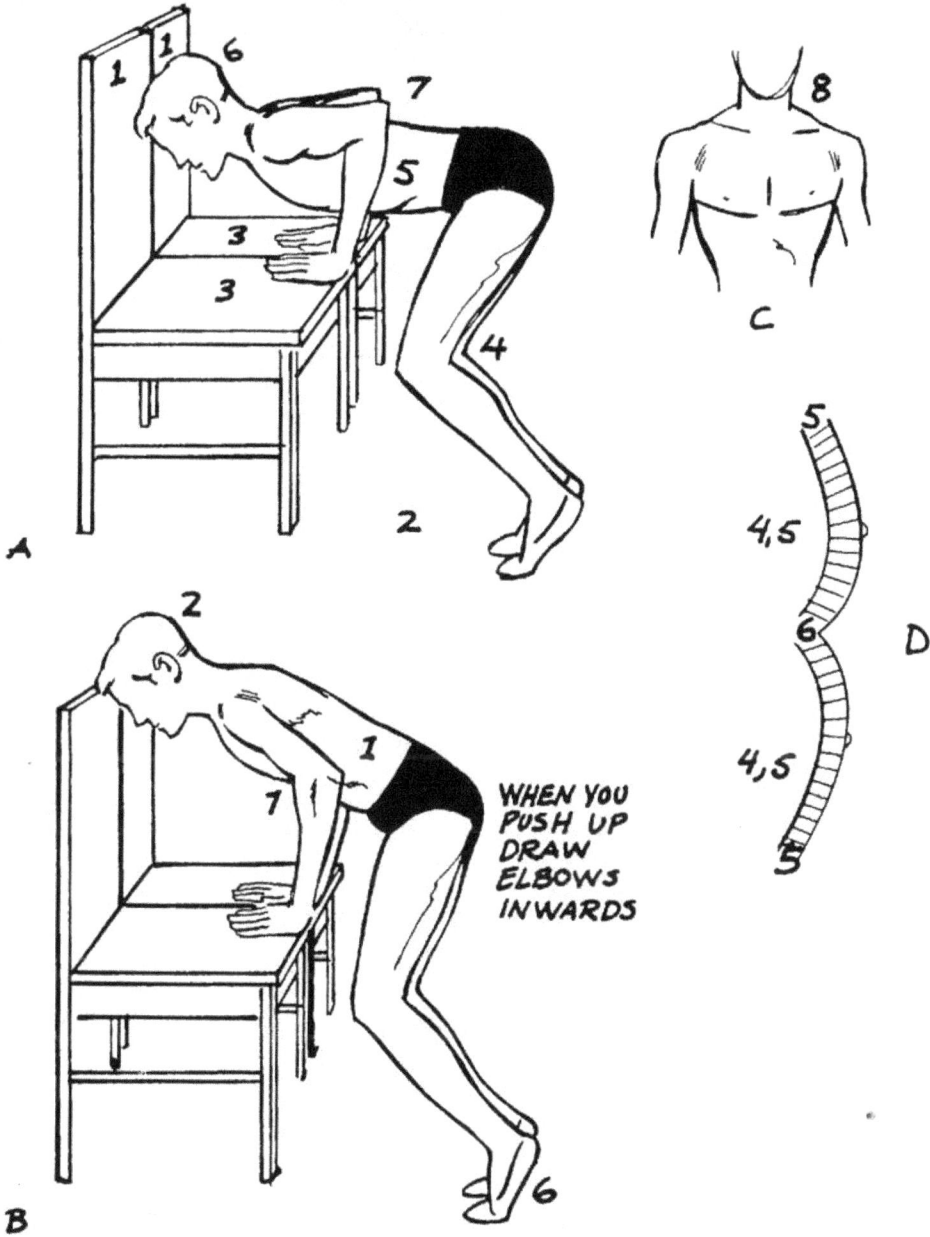

Figure 37
Your Emotion Ouster

How to do this Yoga mov-asana (Figures 37 C,D)

1. Inhale quickly. Then exhale as you
2. Push up your dropped weight about 4 or 5 inches.

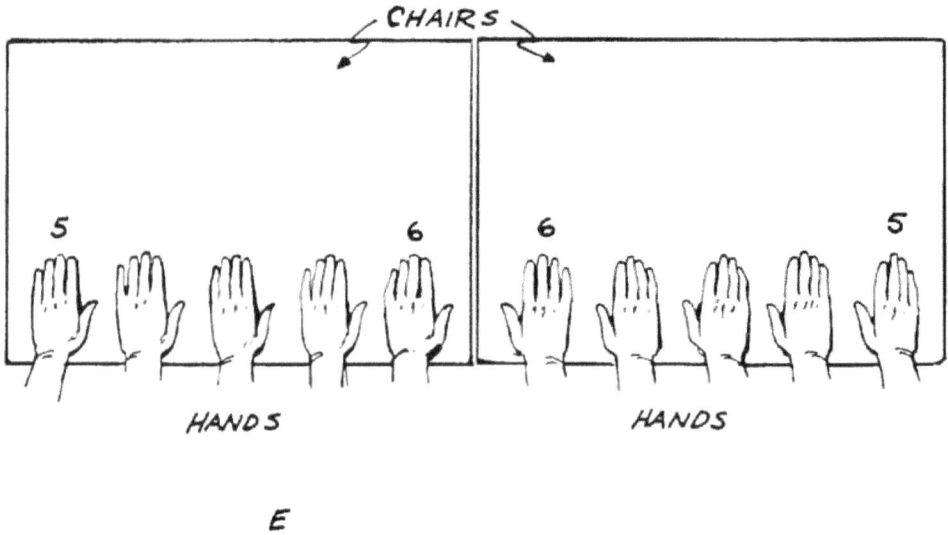

Figure 37, cont.

3. Drop it back and repeat. (Not shown).

4. Bear your weight on your lower chest muscle or breast line (Figure 37 D). Keep elbows close to your body. Now,

5. Draw hands about 1 inch closer before the next repetition (Figures 37 C,D).

6. When you push up, your body rocks back a little on your toes (Figure 37 B).

Frequency: 5 repetitions. Each repetition 1 inch closer, until your hands are about 8 or 10 inches apart, depending upon your height and reach. 2-3 sets (groups of repetitions). 4 times a week.

What Your Emotion Ouster does for you (Figure 37 F)

1. Heightens markedly the lower portion of your chest muscles (or breasts). If you are a woman, with or without a brassiere, your breasts will stand up noticeably.

2. Your heavy "pressing" upon those chair seats with your hands and weight frees you of your volcanic emotions, and so you prevent them from blinding you to a hunch when you receive it.

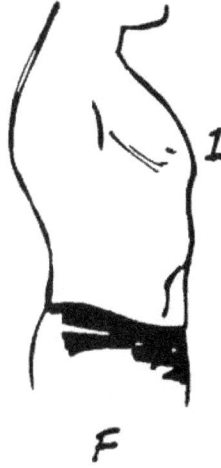

Figure 37, cont.

References

[1]*National Enquirer*, 1972.

[2]Even in physiology, while a freshman in dental school *several decades* before science did, I discovered that brain waves could conrol the mind and the body, and be used for telepathic power, besides! These findings were partly published in 1955, and more fully in 1966 in *Cyclomancy* (West Nyack, New York: Parker Publishing Company, Inc.). Science did not even discover some of them until 1966 (*New Mind, New Body*, Dr Barbara M. Brown). These discoveries are revolutionizing the academic, scientific, economic, healing, social, and military worlds.

12

How Yoga Powers Can Help You
Take Charge in Emergencies

How Yoga Makes You Taller and Strengthens Your Leadership Abilities

Maintaining your height or getting taller makes you look more impressive. It also brings you your best health and longest life and makes you a much stronger leader. The Yogis have known that for thousands of years. The length of your legs does not change once you grow up, but the length of your spine shrinks continually afterwards. By shrinking, it compresses your spinal nerves, which pass through it. That reduces the blood supply to your whole body, from your neck down; weakens the intensity of the sensations your brain receives from your muscles and organs, and of the commands which your brain sends to them. Even if you live long with a shrunken spine, your reflexes are slower, your thinking is less keen, your energy is reduced, and your leadership abilities minimized. By keeping your spine stretched as tall as possible as you advance in years, you don't get "short" with time, and you retain your leadership abilities much longer—perhaps as much as 50 years longer, as do the Yogis.

With Yoga, though, you can even stretch yourself to a taller height than you were originally by straightening your spine still more—and even by stretching the thickness of the spinal discs between your vertebrae. All your mental and physiological functions are correspondingly improved magically, and your leadership abilities strengthened. The Yoga movasana to make you taller is The Sacro-Stretch. Here is how to do it. (Follow Figure 38.)

200

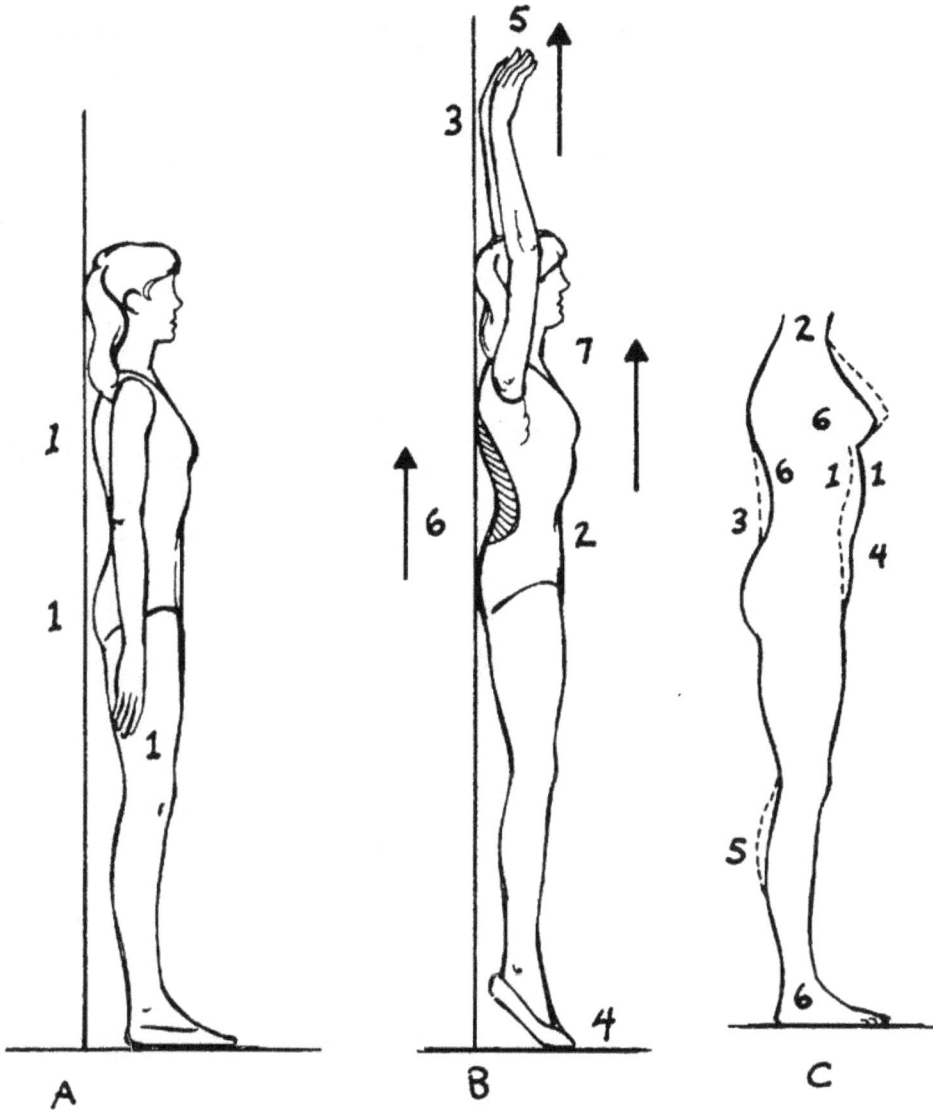

Figure 38
The Sacro-Stretch

The position to assume (Figure 38 A)

    1. Stand straight against a wall or partition, with your arms relaxed at your sides.

How to do this Yoga mov-asana (Figure 38 B)

    2. Inhale deeply, and

3. Raise your arms straight above your head, until the backs of your hands rest against the wall or partition.

4. Rise on your toes. At the same time,

5. Stretch your arms and try to "touch" the ceiling with your fingertips.

6. Stretch your back, too, to the utmost. (Your lower back, especially, will stretch, stimulating your fourth lumbar vertebra, or the vertebra near the base of your spine. The spinal nerve passing between it and your fifth lumbar vertebra below it, stimulates your genitals.)

7. Stretch your neck ceiling-ward. The middle portion of your neck, particularly, will stretch and stimulate the cervical ganglia (nerve cell mass) of the sympathetic nerves in your neck. These nerves, in turn, will stimulate your pituitary gland. Your pituitary gland (if you are a woman) produces hormones that trigger your ovary into action. But whether you are a man or a woman, they encourage your bones to grow, even if at a much more slower pace after passing maturity.

8. Exhale, lower your arms, and reassume your original position.

Frequency: 10 repetitions every morning. 4-5 times a week.

What The Sacro-Stretch mov-asana does for you (Figure 38 C)

1. Expands your rib-box, bringing health to your lungs, and allowing more room for your heart. Your chest (or breasts) are elevated, as a result, and look impressively higher.

2. Increases your height.

3. Firms your sacrospinalis muscles: the muscles of the center of your lower back, which prevent it from sagging.

4. Draws in your waist and wears off fat from the front and sides of it.

5. Fills out the backs of your calves.

6. Fills your lungs and blood with more oxygen. Strengthens your ankles. Relieves the pressure of your vertebrae upon all your spinal nerves, which pass between them, thereby improving your body functions. Tones the extensor muscles of your body, from your neck down to your waist, and the flexor muscles from your waist to your toes, endowing you with the light carriage of youth (Not shown). Increase your sex vigor.

How Lester B. Changed His Whole Physical Aspect for the Better

Lester B. was disappointed with his general appearance. He was in his forties and resented the younger generation for being taller and more streamline-built than he. "Maybe they eat better than I did, and have more leisure!" he sulked. "Just my luck to be born too soon!"

I taught Lester the Sacro-Stretch. In no time he "grew" a half inch, and was still "growing." But the mov-asana also streamlined his figure and made him look about one and one-fourth inches taller! It toned his extensor muscles and drew in his waist, endowing him with the light carriage of youth. Bursting with enthusiasm, Lester felt as if nearly three inches taller. He had *reversed* the years and joined the *new* generation in youth and appearance. He let his hair and sideburns grow longer to fit his new mood. To my own surprise, he fascinated and married a very attractive, wealthy young woman two inches taller than he. In the past she had seen him as being "too old" for her. Now she was smitten with his "youthful maturity."

Mind-Calming Effect of Yoga in a Crisis

A 1972 edition of *Time* magazine reported that "certain kinds of accident rates. . . are influenced by phases of the moon, solar cycles, and other natural phenomena." Scientists, in the same vein, doubt whether all natural phenomena follow strict and universally valid laws. Even your immunity to infection is rhythmic. You have periods of maximum strength or weakness, hours of greater endurance for nervous strain, hours of greater patience, keener perception, greater muscular strength, and even hours of better immunity.[1] It all proves that you are not always in the best state to avoid accidents. At certain times, which cannot easily be determined mathematically, you can avoid accidents more easily than at other times. The margin of escape between safety and accident is unbelievably minute.

The Clutch of Gravity on you is one of those important natural phenomena. Its incessant downward pull can dull your whole muscle-nerve coordination to the degree where you lose enough control over your muscles (even if only temporarily) to fall victim to an accident which you would have otherwise avoided. As a result, you may misjudge time, distance, or place-position. The Yoga mov-asana movement to help you through such an emergency and perhaps save your life is Your Rude Awakener. Here is how to do it. (Follow Figure 39.)

The position to assume (Figure 39 A)

1. Sit straight on a chair or stool with a hard seat.
2. Keep elbows hugging sides, and

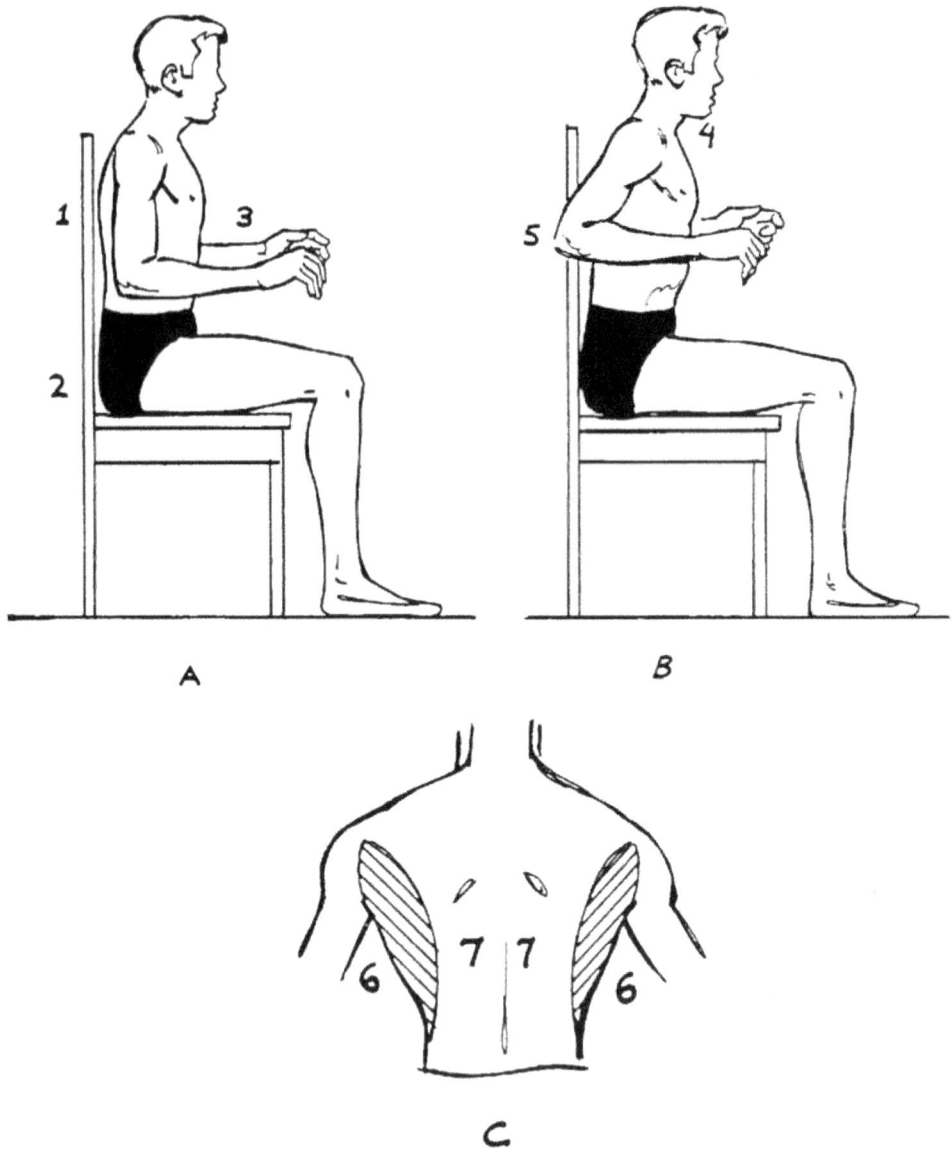

Figure 39
Your Rude Awakener

3. Hold forearms parallel to the floor, palms down.

How to do this Yoga mov-asana (Figure 39 B)

4. Round your shoulder and, *at the same time*,

5. Draw your bent arms suddenly backwards. Hold your back straight.

6. You will feel very firm in the lower part of your back (Figure 39 C-6).

Frequency: 7 repetitions. 2 sets (groups of repetitions). 4-5 times a week.

What Your Rude Awakener does for you (Figure 39 C)

1. V-shapes the upper two-thirds of your back.

2. The sudden firming being at the center of your body, it reflexly stimulates the muscles above and below it. All your muscles, for that reason, are stimulated in part. As a result,

3. All the muscle centers in your brain are jolted awake. You are ready to meet emergencies better and avoid accidents.

How Nicholas D. Saved His Life with a Yoga Mov-asana

Nicholas D. was getting older, like everybody else, and his friends warned him that his reflexes were "slowing down." They cautioned him against doing one thing after another and told him that once he passed 65 he had to "take it easy." Nicholas was inclined to agree with them because he had suffered more accidents than usual in the last few years, even when riding his bicycle in the public park.

Since Nicholas was otherwise in good health, I taught him His Rude Awakener. The sudden firming at the center of his back sent a thrill up his spine and stimulated all his back muscles, up to his neck. It jolted awake the muscle centers in his brain. His mind felt clearer, and his muscles were more responsive to its commands. He felt more daring and more sure of himself. It was as if he had suddenly turned on the power switch to his reflexes.

In a few weeks Nicholas noticed that he handled his bicycle with far more dexterity. He was fortunate because that very day Nicholas turned the wheel just in time to avoid being knocked off his bicycle and perhaps crushed to death. Two months before, he swore, he could not have acted that swiftly. The mov-asana athletically shaped the upper two-thirds of his back. It had already made him *look* from ten to 15 years younger.

Three Yoga Secrets to Cheat Death and Live Decades Longer —and Healthy

With three simple Yoga secrets you can live healthily decades longer. You know them already, but the Yoga secrets reveal them to the utmost. Here they are:

1. Don't smoke. The Yogis have always opposed smoking. So did my medical and dental ancestors and I, although several in the family have been heavy chain-smokers, to the anger and disdain of the others. We insisted that *the very act of smoking* amounted to a suicidal attempt. Now a scientist (Levine) upholds us by showing a *direct link* between smoking and the conditions leading to a heart attack.[1] The very smoking of *one single cigarette*, the researcher found, has a dramatic effect on your blood clotting. The *very act of smoking*, in other words, can cause your blood to clot and bring on a heart attack! Smoking, in addition, has been found to cause *ulcers*.[2] Those who smoke more than 20 cigarettes a day suffer strokes six times more often than do non-smokers.

Note: An investigator at the Harvard School of Public Health reported that cigarette smokers tend to have lower blood pressure, and that the blood pressure jumps when a smoker quits the habit.[3] He failed to explain, however, that tobacco smoking anesthetises your sympathetic nervous system, and that's how it slows down your heart and lowers your blood pressure. By doing so it also diminishes your energy and your daily efficiency. Should your heart suddenly be called upon to meet an emergency, it may not speed up enough to pump much needed blood into your muscles and brain.

2. If you are a man, don't try to lengthen your life with female sex hormones, like estrogen, and big doses of vitamin E. The Yogis opposed using anything from outside the body, except natural food, to better their health, except in emergencies. The female sex hormones, when used in men, have been found in a nationwide study to increase the incidence of cancer, particularly lung cancer.[4] Men using them also suffer more from blood clots. In my own researches I have found that such "drugs" increase the growth of the prostate in men, which could lead to prostate cancer.

And whether you are a man or a woman, avoid "body-building drugs." Athletes, both men and women, often use them to achieve remarkable physical development and trim fat off their hips quickly. With them, muscle men may attain fantastic muscle bulk, and both men and women may perform at their greatest level in competition. These "body-building drugs" are the androgenic-anabolic steroids. They are given in large quantities in many sports nowadays.[5] Since 1954 (the beginning of their wide spread use) I opposed them vigorously and pleaded in vain with aspiring athletes and musclemen to bypass them. Nineteen years later, two of them died of cancer of the colon, a third became severely ill with cancer of the bladder, and a fourth has been hospitalized. Nineteen years later the scientists found that these products *can* severely harm the health and cause certain cancers. They can weaken the heart and shrink the testicles. *Of course*, you can attain faster and more striking physical results by adding such drugs to your diet than with the Yoga mov-asanas alone. But with the mov-asanas you can look stunning *and still* remain healthy all your life. With the "drugs" you can shine for a few years—but probably doom yourself to a comparatively early, terrible, lingering death. It is wiser to leave Nature alone, as the Yogis do. If your body is normal otherwise, put nothing "foreign" into it.

3. Don't drink. The Yogis abstained from all spirited drinks and liquors. So did my medical and dental ancestors, and so did I myself. An expert warns now that alcohol kills and disables more people each year than all other drugs combined![6]

Obey these three Yoga secrets religiously, and you will already cheat death in many different ways and live healthy for decades longer.

How to Prevent Your Brain Center from Building up a Heart Attack

Friedman, a major cardiologist, discovered[7] after 25 years' research that your heart attack is triggered by your brain. If you convert yourself into a hardworking, aggressive perfectionist who never asks for help, can't waste time, trying to succeed at everything you tackle and have no time to play, you are a Type A heart attack prone. If you are such a person, diet won't help you much the cardiologist insists, for at most, it can lower your cholesterol level only by a small fraction. You don't have to be a "worrier," besides, to trigger heart attacks with your brain. You just need to be a person who attacks the challenges of life.

If you *are* such a person, you can use that same driving brain of yours to *defuse* an oncoming attack. You can still attack life and work with determination to achieve your fondest dreams. But instead of letting your emotion brain center go off half-cocked with your single-mindedness, normalize it regularly, preferably every half hour or so, or whenever you feel tense. That will *de*-intensify the excessive stimulations of your fighting sympathetic nervous system on your heart and relax your tensing heart muscles. It will discourage heart attacks from building up in your system and defuse oncoming ones. Certain Yogis are masters at this skill and use it repeatedly to escape death and live remarkably long lives.

To avoid heart attacks, Dr. Friedman advises, "keep cool."[8] That's precisely what the Yogis do. They keep cool by withdrawing the aggressiveness from their sympathetic nervous systems at fixed intervals during their waking hours, and hence preventing the centers for their heart action in their brains from building up to dangerous tensions that can trigger heart attacks.

Defusing an Oncoming Heart Attack with an Appropriate Brain Wave

Another physician, Dr. William S. Kroger of Beverly Hills, California, contends that sexual frustration is often an indirect cause of heart attack. If you are a man, for example, sexual frustration may result when your wife rejects you for "impotency" or for the lack of enough lovemaking skill. If you are a woman, it may result when your husband notices your lessening sex appeal. You are driven, as a result, to escape in overworking and fall victim to fatigue, putting you on the road to an early grave. Doctors from Boston University Medical Center, too, (according to *The New England Journal of Medicine*) advise you to skip your coffee break if you have a weak heart. Dr. Edward Terry Dawson, a staff cardiologist at the Long Island Jewish-Hinsdale Medical Center, at a meeting on "Sex and the Coronary Victim," asserts, though, that sex may be one of the best forms of exercise for heart patients. Speaking for the Yogis, I agree that certain mov-asanas (see Index) strengthen the heart of the heart patient. Adding sex to any kind of physical exercise, though, also adds intense glandular stimulation to the efforts and overworks your heart.

The Yogis prefer to defuse oncoming heart attacks with appropriate brain waves. Recently, several research studies by scientists have supported them. These studies have shown a definite link between brain wave patterns and impending heart attacks. One researcher, Dr. James Birren, director of the University of Southern California Gerontology Center in Los Angeles, found that there was as much blood flowing in a healthy man's brain at 73 as at 25. It was also found, however, that the older man had *slower* brain wave frequencies than younger men.

The secret Yoga mov-asana to defuse an oncoming heart attack with an appropriate brain wave is Your Brain-Wave Accelerator. Here is how to do it.

Your Brain-Wave Accelerator—
for Saving Your Heart

1. Every half hour or so during your hectic day, suddenly drop your jaw. Simultaneously, relax the muscles in the backs of your shoulders (your trapezius muscles) by rotating your shoulders in full circles. Your jaw and shoulder muscles tense when your mind works intently. At such times you may find yourself biting on your teeth and feeling tight and uncomfortable in the backs of your shoulders. You are chewing up your "enemy," in other words.

Reflexly, your heart is ready to speed up and rush more blood to your fighting muscles. It is not a relaxed heart then. It is, instead, like a crouching cat, ready to spring into furious action. The tension of this suppressed waiting whips your heart muscle into a state in which it can literally go into a spasm. Even your brain waves could reveal this early sign of heart danger, for heart disease can cause your brain waves to slow down. It explains why older men have slower brain wave frequencies than younger men (Birren).[9]

2. To counteract the building up of this spasm tendency on your heart, to repeat, every half hour during your hectic day drop your jaw and rotate your shoulders in circles, for about ten seconds. By the end of the ten seconds the brain wave of your tensed heart will alter into that of your heart when it functions normally. *This* is the appropriate brain wave for you to use to defuse an oncoming heart attack in you. Practice a little and get the exact "feel" of this heart-relaxed brain wave. Be able to throw yourself into it instantly whenever you wish. With it you will postpone significantly your possibilities of suffering a heart attack by defusing it with this brain wave at once whenever you sense it coming on.

Note: I maintain, in fact, (and in the years to come, science will again uphold me and prove me to be far ahead of my time) that being a Type A heart attack prone type will *not* trigger a heart attack at all—if you engage faithfully in simple movements and scientific mov-asanas like those described in my books *Somo-Psychic Power: Using Its Miracle Forces For a Fabulous New Life*, *Yoga For Men Only*, or this very book. I have proof of that in myself and in others who did them. These exercises and mov-asanas normalize the tensions of my research and writing and keep me in top heart shape.[10] Being a so-called Type A "heart attack" type of personality, indeed, is a tremendous help to achieve your goals. It increases your efficiency beyond measure. I will never alter myself into a different type of person, but will retain my remarkable heart with it and live up to between 125 and 250 years! *Let's do it together!*

The Yoga Secrets to Control Sciatic Trouble

Sciatic trouble usually indicates that the different bones in your hip-joint are not articulating with precision. Your sciatic nerve (one in each hip) passes between these bones, all the way from your spine down to your toes. When you suffer from sciatic trouble this nerve is pinched by your incorrectly-articulating hip-joint and causes a number of discomforts in you. They may range all the way from insufferable pain in that hip or inability to walk to numbness anywhere from your hips down to your toes. The purpose of this book is not to keep you from seeing your doctor, osteopath, or chiropractor when you suffer from any trouble. But it can show you how to prevent or heal trouble, such as in the following section. (Follow Figure 40.)

How to Prevent Sciatic Trouble

1. Don't run *downhill*. You only jolt your back at every down step, over-

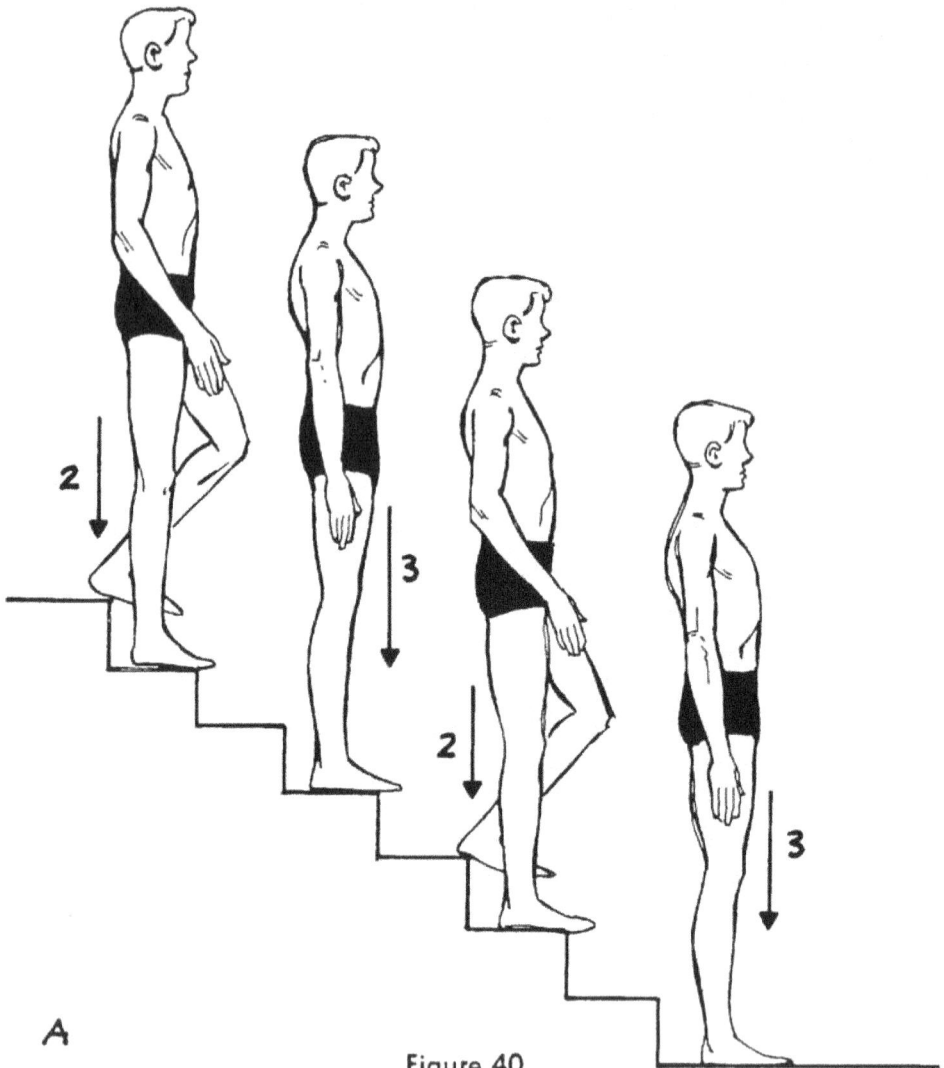

Figure 40
For Sciatic Trouble

compress the intervertebral discs in your back, and ram your femur (your thigh bone) into your hip-joint with arthritis-creating power.

2. Don't climb down from a too-high elevation upon one leg at a time, with your body straight and facing front. Go down nearly turning sideways, instead, and rest your weight on one hand first, such as by placing that hand upon the ground where you are standing (Figure 40 A). Then let one leg down upon the lower elevation, with your trunk leaning over your hands to ease the weight (Figure 40 A). In that way your descending leg carries little of your body weight on it. That prevents the jolting force of descending from ramming your thigh bone into your hip-joint and pushing one of the three closely-fitting bones that comprise it out of joint. Then lower your second leg to the *same step as* or level with the first.

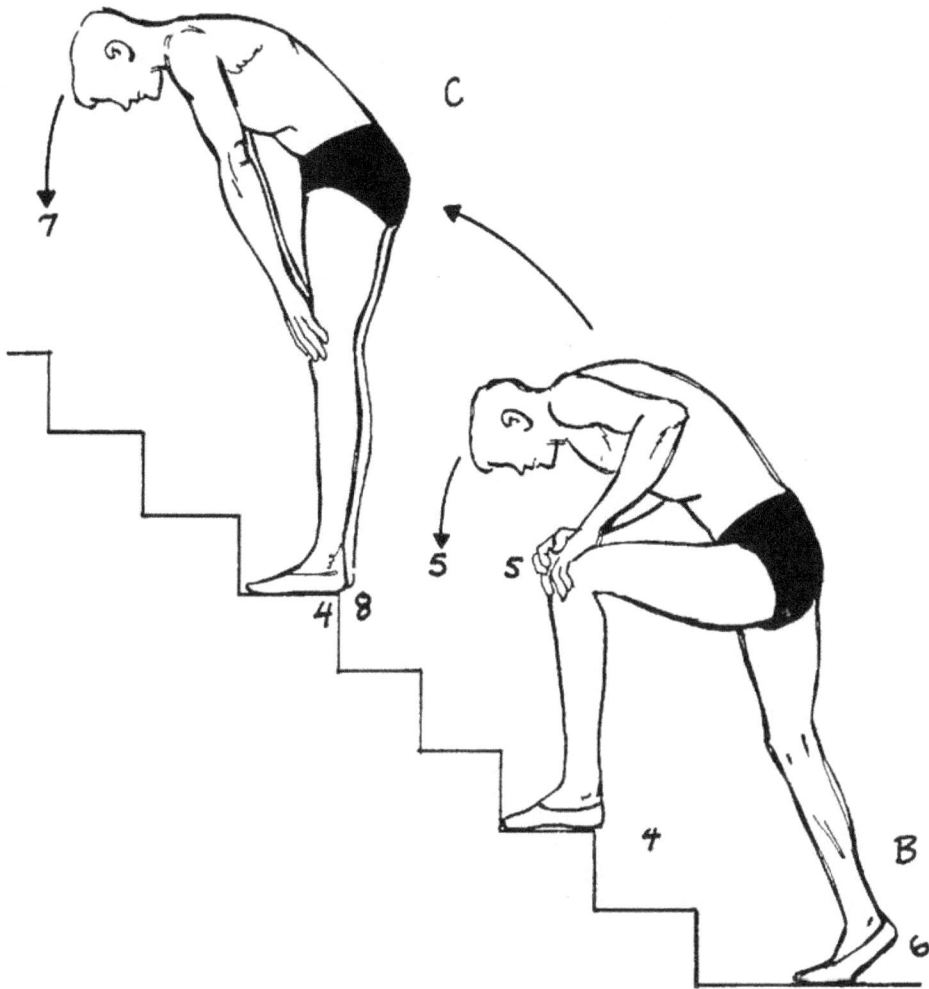

Figure 40, cont.

3. Don't neglect climbing stairs every day, or climbing a hilly place if you are outdoors. It keeps the ligaments that bind your hip-joint strong. Once these ligaments weaken from lack of exercise or proper use, your hip-joint is easily subluxated (partially dislocated), causing you sciatic pain and incapacity. Climb the stairs by two's, and if you are tall, by three's. If you have no stairs, or if they are too short for a "good" climbing, and if you can't climb outdoors, do The Torso Push (page 37). Do this mov-asana, anywhere, to strengthen your hip-joints. Bicycling also strengthens them when you pedal in high gear, although it really seems to use your knees more than your hips. But to ride it daily might be inconvenient and unsafe after work. Jogging does not strengthen your hips enough because you don't have to bend your knees deeply for it. Sprinting, in that regard, is better, especially if you sprint *up* a hill.

4. Don't neglect these preventive measures. To suffer from hip-trouble, particularly as you advance in years, as occurs to so many people, is to condemn

yourself to the wheelchair during the last years of your life, or to stumble around on a cane, *if* you can. Weak hips can cause you to fall and break them and confine you to bed, thus threatening you with blood clots.

How to Help Overcome Sciatic Trouble

1. Do The Torso Push, (page 37) to strengthen and normalize the lengths of the overstretched ligaments around your afflicted hip-joint and keep the bones that comprise your hip-joint in place. Do one set several times a day when your stomach is empty, up to a total of 25 to 50 repetitions for a few days, to help prevent a recurrence of the subluxation (partial dislocation). Also observe these cautions:

2. Climb *down* stairs or down the edges of sidewalks on your "sciatic" side. Climb down gently, step-by-step, always leading *with that* bad leg (Figure 40 A) and on the *flat* of the *whole foot*.

3. Bring your "good leg" down to it at each step. (Follow Figure 40.) And keep the knee of your "sciatic" side *straight*, both when you are climbing down with that leg, and when you are bringing down the "good leg" to it.

That maneuver keeps your body weight off your "sciatic" joint and throws it, instead, upon the shaft of the *straightened* bone of that leg. Keep your "sciatic" joint fixed, in other words, to prevent it from being used until it heals.

4. When you climb *up* stairs or upon sidewalks, place the *whole foot* of your "sciatic" side upon the higher step, not just the ball of the foot (Figure 40 B).

5. Then rest your hands near the knee of that thigh and lean your weight forward on them.

6. Push up your body with the foot of your "good" side, and

7. Continue leaning forward (Figure 40 B) until

8. You bring that foot up to the foot of your "sciatic" side.

9. After doing The Torso Push (as you were instructed in Number 1 of this list) for your sciatic trouble, you might feel alarmingly stiff next morning and fear that you have gotten worse. This mov-asana will have stretched the facial (thick fibrous) sheaths surrounding your hips, and these are extensive. Stiffness should go that morning after three more sets of this mov-asana, or diminish so much that you feel like a totally different person. Continue doing Numbers 2 to 9 and you will be astonished at how speedily you continue freeing yourself from the condition. In three days or less it should be gone or be nearly gone so that you hardly remember it.

The Yoga Secret to Build Yourself up Fast

If you are a man you may want to enlarge your shoulders, chest, arms, back, thighs, calves, and other muscles, fast. You may want to look and feel Herculean in your clothes and in a bathing suit, and stand out in the crowd. If you are young enough you may desire to compete in physique contests—and win. (In this, though, you are now also required to compete lifting weights to win, so you would have to practice with them, too.) If you are too thin or shapeless a woman, you may wish to fill out your breasts, round out your shoulders, and shape your legs—all in a hurry.

The Yogis have the answer. This is the procedure for you:

1. Find in the Index the part of your body which you want to enlarge fast. Do, particularly, the mov-asanas listed under arms, back, bulk, chest, neck-shoulder lines, shoulders, and thighs. (For thighs, still use both of them at the same time, but with three sets of repetitions, done strenuously.)

2. Turn to the page or pages indicated for the best mov-asana (or mov-asanas) to achieve that goal.

3. If you are doing mov-asanas five days a week, do those you have selected in Number 2 with the following number of repetitions:

First day: 4 alternating repetitions with each arm for each set. (To be explained later.)

Second day: 10 repetitions with each arm for each set.

Third day: 4 alternating repetitions with each arm for each set.

Fourth day: 10 repetitions with both arms at the same time for each set.

Fifth day: 1 alternating repetition with each arm for each set.

Sixth and seventh day: Rest, or do abdominal mov-asanas alone to keep your waist getting trimmer.

How to get the best results:

4. The fast "get big" days are the first, third, and fifth. You do less repetitions then because you do them with *much more power* than on the second and fourth days. This is how you do them on the first, third, and fifth days:

(a) Instead of doing them with both arms at the same time, as described in the book,

(b) Drop all your weight on one arm for each repetition. Your body will twist naturally as you do so, towards that arm.

5. By dropping all your weight on one arm at a time, all the muscle fibers of that arm are thrown into contraction at the same time, triggering their maximum growth. Its bones, ligaments, tendons, and sinews are affected likewise, all contributing to its speedy maximum growth in size and power.

6. Resist, also, the effort of that one arm *more* with the rest of your body, as described in the book for each mov-asana.

7. Since, as stated in 4A, your body twists naturally to drop your whole weight on the arm being exercised, this twist contracts the sides of your waist to a

boil-like tightness. Your abdominal obliques, as a result, are drawn in deep and reduce the girth of your waist to an astonishing degree. You thereby acquire massive size (or become much bigger, if you are a woman) in the chest (or breasts), shoulders, arms, back. But, at the same time, your waist shrinks to a cartoon-like nothingness. . . even if you don't feel the tightness.

The wisest plan to get the best results

8. Do the repetitions of days 1, 3, and 5 one limb at a time, that is, do one repetition with your left arm, and then one with your right. That, in Step 3, amounts to *one* repetition. So, when you perform the number of repetitions called for in the first, third, and fifth days in 3, do each repetition alternately with each arm.

9. Your greatest bulk is gained from your fifth day workout, the day when you do only one repetition with each arm. Throw your whole weight on the arm being exercised and resist (as described in the mov-asana) to the utmost degree. At the end of its repetition the arm should feel that it can't make another one and should retain just enough strength to balance your body while you make one repetition with the opposite arm.

Then stand up, breathing heavily, and walk for a half minute to rest before doing the next one repetition set. At the end of the three sets (or whatever number is called for in the book for that mov-asana) the muscles being exercised should feel larger and larger, for they will be engorged with nutrient-carrying blood.

10. At the end of the fifth day workout you will need the sixth and seventh days to rest and regain your full strength. Those two days, too, will permit the tissues of your muscles, bones, ligaments and sinews to grow faster to handle the extra strain.

11. After three months on such a program, you will be fantastically bigger. But you will already notice significant gains from the very first week. Within three months you could add from ten to 30 lbs. of solid muscle to your body, depending on your natural size and physique type, and constrict your waist to the minuteness of a starving teen-ager.

And you don't need extra or different kinds of food preparations, unusual apparatus, or pills of any kind. Your body will respond naturally to the extra calls for more effort and will grow the necessary additional tissue.[11]

An effective compromise

12. If you can spare only three after-work periods a week for the mov-asanas instead of five, then do the first, third, and fifth days as described in 3, and rest from exercise on the days in between. You will then require about one-third longer to attain your physical goal and won't enjoy as trim a muscular delineation as the five-day program. This may satisfy you if you are a woman and wish only to "fill out" more. But if you are a man you will need the in between

days with their higher repetitions to look your most impressive.

This is how to make up that loss. After four months, change for a month of three day workouts of ten repetitions for each mov-asana with both arms at the same time, as described in the book. It will maintain the size gains you have made, and also reward you with trim muscle definition. Performing the mov-asanas with both arms at the same time, too, carves a deep center groove on your chest and in the middle thirds of your back and abdomen. Without these festoons your figure will not appear at its best. With them, though, you will reach your peak of physical perfection. So, if you are unable to adopt a five-day after work mov-asana program, attain your goal to "get big" fast with a three-day program, even if it takes a little longer.

Important: Powerful (and bulkier) thigh muscles slow you down when you jog on a level surface. But they speed you up when you climb stairs or run up a hill. You need more powerful and bigger thigh muscles then, which won't tire so easily from the added muscular effort. It has been proved, besides, that running up a hill (or stairs by two's) rewards you with a much stronger heart than running on a level surface.

Afterword

You have now completed *Yoga Secrets for Extraordinary Health and Long Life*. You found, in its pages, the most fantastic revelation of natural health and longevity secrets in the history of human health. Use them to attain the miracle health and long life that so many Yogis have. Turn to the front of the book, to the Contents, to find the pages of specific material. Follow the thorough instructions carefully and stop being victimized by health ignorance and superstition. Be born again into your youthful prime, and stay that way until the end.

More Scientific Support of the Remarkable Truths of My Secrets

A 10-year test by California investigators checked the health of a population of 7,000 in a typical community against their style of living (1974). They tested eight specific habits. The results of their tests showed that the healthiest citizens believe in following the "exact" health formulas which I myself have believed and practiced regularly since I was 24. I taught the first six of them since 1954. I added the seventh to my teachings since 1957, and the eighth since 1960. In brief, I taught all eight of them from 14 to 20 years before science even tested and accepted such as the best health formulas. These are my magic 8 health formulas.

1. A good night's sleep (seven to eight hours)[12]

2. Three square meals a day (no more, no less)[13]

3. Regular exercise[14]

4. No smoking[15]

5. Drink moderately or not at all[16]

6. Maintain reasonably good weight for height[17]

7. Eat breakfast almost every day[18]

8. Don't eat between meals[19]

The people tested who followed formulas 7 and 8 had remarkably better health than those who skipped breakfast and ate between meals.

Dr. Lester Breslow, Dean of the School of Public Health of the University of California, concluded from the results of his tests that there was a conclusive relation between good health habits and the status of physical health. [20]

That's why this book brings you the secrets of extraordinary health and long life. *Solar Diet* (now out of print) was obviously about 20 years ahead of its time. This book, I predict, also is.

References

[1]Dr. Peter H. Levine, university researcher of Tufts New England Medical Center, 1974.

[2]Dr. Philip A. Wolf, American Academy of Neurology, 1974.

[3]Dr. Jeremiah Stamler, scientist, Northwestern University; and a member of the research team composed of scientists from 53 medical centers.

[4]A team of scientists from five scientific departments of U.S. universities; *Lancet*, the authoritative British medical journal.

[5]Dr. Fort, a former consultant on drug abuse to the World Health Organization.

[6]Dr. Meyer Friedman, major San Francisco cardiologist, after 25 years of research.

[7]*Ibid*.

[8]*Ibid*.

[9]Dr. James Birren, director of the University of Southern California Gerontology Center in Los Angeles. From research with the Federal Aviation Agency (FAA).

[10]As far back as Nov. 30, 1935, I wrote to a personal friend, "It's always good to follow some kind of exercise systematically. Several times when I feel

depressed, or can't take a workout, and solve a writing problem (or am under anxiety or tension) I take a workout, and the answer is soon before me.'' That discovery puts me again over 40 years ahead of science, for science has not yet agreed with me. But eventually, it will.

[11]Ken Norton, the famous heavyweight boxer whose outstanding physical development brought him the movie role in *Mandigo*, has never lifted weights. He has just done "natural exercises."

[12]Frank Rudolph Young, *Solar Diet* (West Nyack, N.Y.: Parker Publishing Company, Inc., 1954), p. 11.

[13]*Ibid.*, pp. 12, 13, 17, 22, 23, 24.

[14]Frank Rudolph Young, *Yoga For Men Only* (West Nyack, N.Y.: Parker Publishing Company, Inc., 1969).

[15]Young, *Solar Diet*. A study announced on WBBM radio, October 11, 1975, found that men who smoke 2 packs of cigarettes a day, shorten their lives by 15 years. Women, by 20 years. This is considerably more than smaller figures circulated before.

[16]*Ibid.*

[17]*Ibid.*

[18]*Ibid.*, pp. 12, 18, 22.

[19]*Ibid.*

[20]STILL FURTHER SCIENTIFIC CONFIRMATION. Dr. Breslow, furthermore announced in October, 1975, that a man of 55, besides has the same "physical status" as one from *25 to 30 years younger* who follows less than 2 of the magic health rules. Between 1900 and 1970, he noted by comparison, modern medicine has added *only 3 years* to the average American's life. This, Dr. Breslow specified, includes the advances of surgery, antibiotics, anesthesia, as well as all the social changes that have been brought about during that period. Now you know why I look—and feel—and *am* but "half" my age. This is another historic scientific "acknowledgement" of the truth and effectiveness of my far-ahead-of-my-times discoveries. My readers and students who have been taught these 8 magic formulas from 14 to 20 years ahead of science's proofs, have profited from them *beyond measure*—for you *can't buy health* and *many more years of life* with *money*. This book contains, in addition, *hundreds of secrets beyond these* which *you yourself* can put to work right now—perhaps another 20 years before science "acknowledges" them, and thereby *add many more years of health and life* to yourself than you will be able to add that much later.

Index

L

M

N

O

P

Q

R

S

Y

OTHER INSPIRATIONAL AND METAPHYSICAL BOOKS

FROM PARKER PUBLISHING COMPANY

THAT YOU WON'T WANT TO MISS!

- Amazing Laws of Cosmic Mind Power, Joseph Murphy

- The cosmic Energizer: Miracle Power of the Universe, Joseph Murphy

- The Cosmic Power Within You, Joseph Murphy

- Helping Yourself with White Witchcraft, Al G. Manning

- Infinite Power for Richer Living, Joseph Murphy

- Life Beyond Life: The Evidence for Reincarnation, Hans Holzer

- Miracle Power for Infinite Riches, Joseph Murphy

- The Mystic Path to Cosmic Power, Vernon Howard

- The Power of Miracle Metaphysics, Robert B. Stone

- The Power of Your Subconscious Mind, Joseph Murphy

- Prosperity and the Healing Power of prayer, B. Turner

- Psychic Energy: How to Change the Desires into Realities, Joseph Weed

- Psychic Perception, Joseph Murphy

- Psychico-Pictography: The New Way to Use the Miracle Power of your Mind, Vernon Howard

- Secrets of the I-Ching, Joseph Murphy

- Secrets of Mental Magic, Vernon Howard

- Telecult Power: Amazing New Way to Psychic and Occult Wonders, Reese P. Dubin

- Wisdom of Your Subconscious Mind, John K. Williams

- Wisdon of the Mystic Masters, Joseph Weed

- Your Infinite Power to Be Rich, Joseph Murphy

BUY THEM AT

www.parkerpub.co

OR YOUR LOCAL BOOKSTORE

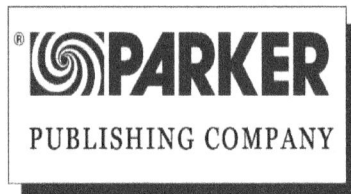

⑉PARKER
PUBLISHING COMPANY

Get Published!

'Everyone has something they know well or can do well. And when a person has a skill, there's always going to be someone willing to pay for it."

parkerpub.co

Parker Publishing Company helps authors publish more titles. So whether you're writing a metaphysical, romance novel, a historical fiction, a mystery, action or suspense story, poetry, business, a children's book, or any other writer, we can help you reach your publishing goals.

Since 1960 we've offered a unique publishing experience to Authors, all over the world. Parker Publishing Company wants to help new authors in all aspects of publishing. The editing, marketing, multi-media design and copyright production and enforcement. From eBooks, Paperback, Hardcovers to Audiobooks can be produced in small volumes and offered to the public.

Besides telling a story, a book is a promotional tool. A book can be likened to a powerful business card since most people won't throw it out. Authoring a book can give you credibility and status, enabling you to charge more for your services.

Your writing will reach more than 20,000 retail accounts worldwide (chains, independents, specialty stores, and libraries). Our United States, Australia and United Kingdom-based sales teams work with clients all over the world through our broad distribution channel partners. For more information please contact us at **www.parkerpub.co**

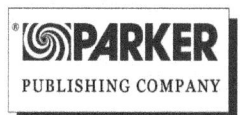

ⓇⓈ❙PARKER
PUBLISHING COMPANY

NOTES

NOTES

NOTES

NOTES

NOTES

NOTES

NOTES

NOTES

NOTES

NOTES

NOTES

www.ingramcontent.com/pod-product-compliance
Lightning Source LLC
Chambersburg PA
CBHW080758300326
41914CB00055B/945